Red cell deformability and filterability

AF850147

Groupe de Travail sur la
Filtration Érythrocytaire

The Royal Society
of Medicine

DEVELOPMENTS IN HEMATOLOGY AND IMMUNOLOGY

Already published in this series:

Lijnen, H.R., Collen, D. and Verstraete, M., eds: Synthetic Substrates in Clinical Blood Coagulation Assays. 1980. ISBN 90-247-2409-0

Smit Sibinga, C.Th., Das, P.C. and Forfar, J.O., eds: Paediatrics and Blood Transfusion. 1982. ISBN 90-247-2619-0

Fabris, N., ed: Immunology and Ageing. 1982. ISBN 90-247-2640-9

Hornstra, G.: Dietary Fats, Prostanoids and Arterial Thrombosis. 1982. ISBN 90-247-2667-0

Smit Sibinga, C.Th., Das, P.C. and Loghem, van J.J., eds: Blood Transfusion and Problems of Bleeding. 1982. ISBN 90-247-3058-9

RED CELL DEFORMABILITY AND FILTERABILITY

Proceedings of the second workshop held in London, 23 and 24 September 1982 under the auspices of The Royal Society of Medicine and the Groupe de Travail sur la Filtration Erythrocytaire

Edited by
JOHN DORMANDY, M.D., F.R.C.S.
St. James' and St. George's Hospitals, London

1983 **MARTINUS NIJHOFF PUBLISHERS**
a member of the KLUWER ACADEMIC PUBLISHERS GROUP
BOSTON / THE HAGUE / DORDRECHT / LANCASTER

Distributors

for the United States and Canada: Kluwer Boston, Inc., 190 Old Derby Street, Hingham, MA 02043, U.S.A.
for all other countries: Kluwer Academic Publishers Group, Distribution Center, P.O. Box 322, 3300 AH Dordrecht, The Netherlands

Library of Congress Cataloging in Publication Data

Main entry under title:

Red cell deformability and filterability.

(Developments in hematology and immunology ;)
"Proceedings of the Second London Workshop on Red Cell Filtration and Deformability"--Pref.
1. Erythrocytes--Congresses. 2. Rheology (Biology)--Congresses. I. Dormandy, J. A. II. Royal Society of Medicine (Great Britain) III. Groupe de travail sur la filtration érythrocytaire. IV. London Workshop on Red Cell Filtration and Deformability (2nd : 1982) V. Series. [DNLM: 1. Erythrocytes, Abnormal--Congresses. 2. Ultrafiltration--Congresses. 3. Blood--Congresses. W1 DE997VZK v.6 / WH 150 R305 1982]
QP96.R315 1983 616.07'561 83-7281

ISBN-13: 978-94-009-6728-1 e-ISBN-13: 978-94-009-6726-7
DOI: 10.1007/978-94-009-6726-7

The organization of this second London workshop and the publication of the proceedings have been made possible by financial support from Hoechst. The help of Ms. Barbara Komoniewska BA, conference secretary of the Royal Society of Medicine, in preparing the texts and discussions for publication is gratefully acknowledged.

Copyright

© 1983 by Martinus Nijhoff Publishers, Boston.
Softcover reprint of the hardcover 1st edition 1983

All rights reserved. No part of this publication may be reproduced, stored in a retrieval system, or transmitted in any form or by any means, mechanical, photocopying, recording, or otherwise, without the prior written permission of the publishers,
Martinus Nijhoff Publishers, 190 Old Derby Street, Hingham, MA 02043, U.S.A.

Preface

This book is an edited verbatim account of the proceedings of the Second London Workshop on Red Cell Filtration and Deformability, organised jointly by the Royal Society of Medicine and the Groupe de Travail sur la Filtration Erythrocytaire. The first such London Workshop was held on the occasion of the Second European Conference on Clinical Haemorheology in 1981 and its conclusions were published in an abbreviated form. The interest in blood filtration as a technique for assessing red cell deformability has continued to increase and there are now several hundred centres around the world using some form of filtration. It was, therefore, felt that the informal detailed discussions held by a small invited group of experts from many countries would be of more general interest and therefore worth publishing. This has been made possible by the continued interest and generous support of Hoechst.

Spontaneous open discussion rather than formal presentations has been the hallmark of these workshops, with precirculation of all scientific data to the participants. We have attempted to preserve this flavour in editing the transcript of the proceedings. This, together with our anxiety for rapid publication, may have resulted in a less than finely polished text which may contain some inaccuracies. The topics discussed were loosely structured into eight sessions, outlined in the accompanying programme. At the end of each session the discussion was summarised by one of us, who was also primarily responsible for editing the transcript of each session before publication. All the sessions were chaired by Peter Gaehtgens. Although every attempt was made within the constraints of available time to eliminate inaccuracies or errors, any remaining in the text must be my responsibility.

It is important for the further effective functioning of these workshops that it should be made aware of all new developments in the field of red cell filtration as well as other alternative new techniques for the assessment of red cell deformability practical for clinical use. We would therefore like to invite any of our colleagues with relevant information to get in touch with the secretariat (Barbara Komoniewska BA, The Royal Society of Medicine, 1 Wimpole Street, London 81M 8AE, U.K.). We would welcome the opportunity of looking at any new information and, if the author wishes, to consider it at our next meeting in October 1983. The information would, of course, not be published or referred to in any form whatsoever without the author's specific permission. We would also very much welcome any comment on the views and information contained in these proceedings. It is the aim of these workshops to try to co-ordinate, evaluate and help the development of this rapidly expanding field.

John Dormandy

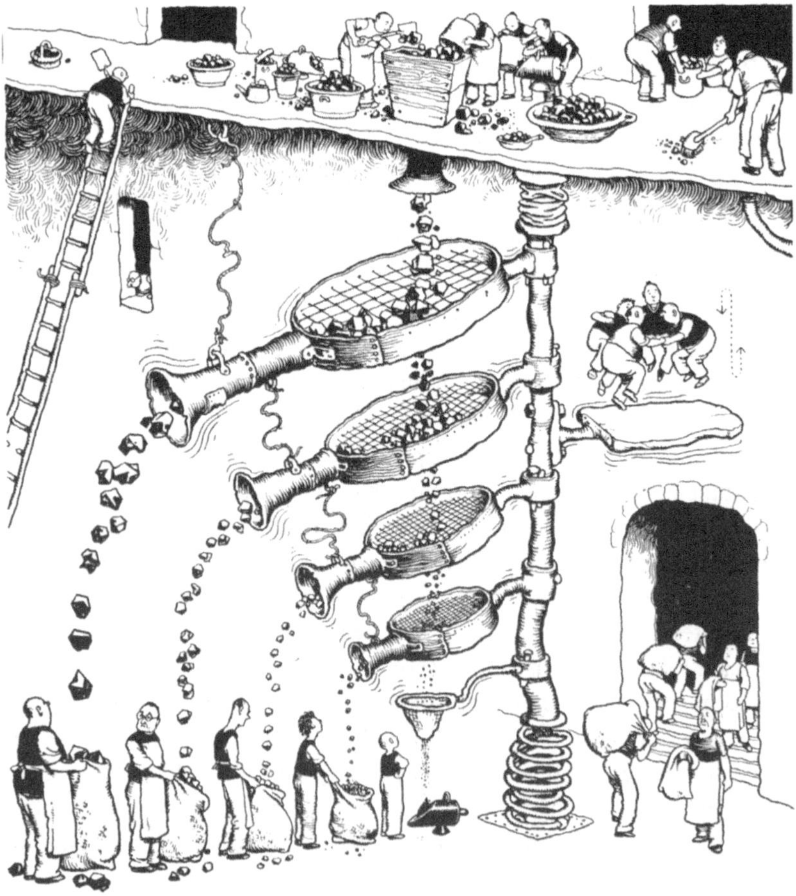

Coke Grading*

* Reproduced from *The Gentle Art of Advertising* by W. Heath Robinson, published by Gerald Duckworth & Co Ltd, London 1979, p. 88.

Contents

List of participants

Dr Adrian Barnes (A.B.)
Barnet General Hospital, Wellhouse Lane, Barnet EN5 3DJ, UK

Mr Peter Buchan (P.B.)
St James' University Hospital, Beckett Street, Leeds LS9 7TF, UK

Professor Shu Chien (S.C.)
Physiology Department, Columbia University College of Physicians and Surgeons, 630 S. 168th Street, New York, USA

Mr John Dormandy (J.D.)
St James' Hospital, Sarsfeld Road, London SW12 8HW, UK

Professor Albrecht Ehrly (A.E.)
Universitätskliniken, Frankfurt am Main 70, Federal Republic of Germany

Professor Sandro Forconi (S.F.)
Istituto di Patologia Speciale Medica, Universita di Siena, Istituti Clinici, Viale Bracci, 53100 Siena, Italy

Professor Peter Gaehtgens (P.G.)
Freie Universität Berlin, Arminallee 22, D-1000 Berlin 33

Professor Maxime Hanss (M.H.)
Université Paris Nord, UER Experimentale, 74 Rue Marcel Cachin, 9300 Bobigny, France

Dr Irene Juhan (I.J.)
Laboratoire Central d'Hématologie, Hôpital de la Timoni, 13385 Marseille

Professor Pierre Leblond (P.L.)
Department of Medicine, Hospital du Saint-Sacrement, 1050 Chemin Ste-Foy, Quebec G1S 4L8, Canada

Dr Gordon Lowe (G.L.)
Department of Medicine, Glasgow Royal Infirmary Glasgow G4 OSF, UK

Dr Georges Marcel (G.A.M.)
Laboratoires Hoechst, 3 Av. du General de Gaulle, 92800 Puteaux, France

Professor Herbert Meiselman (H.M.)
USC School of Medicine, 2025 Zonal Avenue (126 Mudd), Los Angeles, CA 90033, USA

Professor Holger Schmid-Schönbein (H.S-S.)
Abteilung Physiologie, Medizinische Fakultät, Rheinisch-Westfälische Technische Hochschule, Neuklinikum, Forckenbeckstrasse, Aachen, Federal Republic of Germany

Professor Richard Skalak (R.S.)
Bioengineering Institute, Columbia University, 610 Seeley W. Mudd Building, New York, NY 10027, USA

Professor Jean-Francois Stoltz (JF.S.)
Centre Regional de Transfusion Sanguine, Brabois 54500, Vandoeuvre-les-Nancy, France

Professor John Stuart (J.S.)
Department of Haematology, The Medical School, Vincent Drive, Birmingham B15 2TJ, UK

Professor Paul Teitel (P.T.)
Physiology Department, Rheinisch-Westfälische Technische Hochschule, Neuklinikum, Forckenbeckstrasse, Aachen, Federal Republic of Germany

Preface

This book is an edited verbatim account of the proceedings of the Second London Workshop on Red Cell Filtration and Deformability, organised jointly by the Royal Society of Medicine and the Groupe de Travail sur la Filtration Erythrocytaire. The first such London Workshop was held on the occasion of the Second European Conference on Clinical Haemorheology in 1981 and its conclusions were published in an abbreviated form. The interest in blood filtration as a technique for assessing red cell deformability has continued to increase and there are now several hundred centres around the world using some form of filtration. It was, therefore, felt that the informal detailed discussions held by a small invited group of experts from many countries would be of more general interest and therefore worth publishing. This has been made possible by the continued interest and generous support of Hoechst.

Spontaneous open discussion rather than formal presentations has been the hallmark of these workshops, with precirculation of all scientific data to the participants. We have attempted to preserve this flavour in editing the transcript of the proceedings. This, together with our anxiety for rapid publication, may have resulted in a less than finely polished text which may contain some inaccuracies. The topics discussed were loosely structured into eight sessions, outlined in the accompanying programme. At the end of each session the discussion was summarised by one of us, who was also primarily responsible for editing the transcript of each session before publication. All the sessions were chaired by Peter Gaehtgens. Although every attempt was made within the constraints of available time to eliminate inaccuracies or errors, any remaining in the text must be my responsibility.

It is important for the further effective functioning of these workshops that it should be made aware of all new developments in the field of red cell filtration as well as other alternative new techniques for the assessment of red cell deformability practical for clinical use. We would therefore like to invite any of our colleagues with relevant information to get in touch with the secretariat (Barbara Komoniewska BA, The Royal Society of Medicine, 1 Wimpole Street, London 81M 8AE, U.K.). We would welcome the opportunity of looking at any new information and, if the author wishes, to consider it at our next meeting in October 1983. The information would, of course, not be published or referred to in any form whatsoever without the author's specific permission. We would also very much welcome any comment on the views and information contained in these proceedings. It is the aim of these workshops to try to co-ordinate, evaluate and help the development of this rapidly expanding field.

John Dormandy

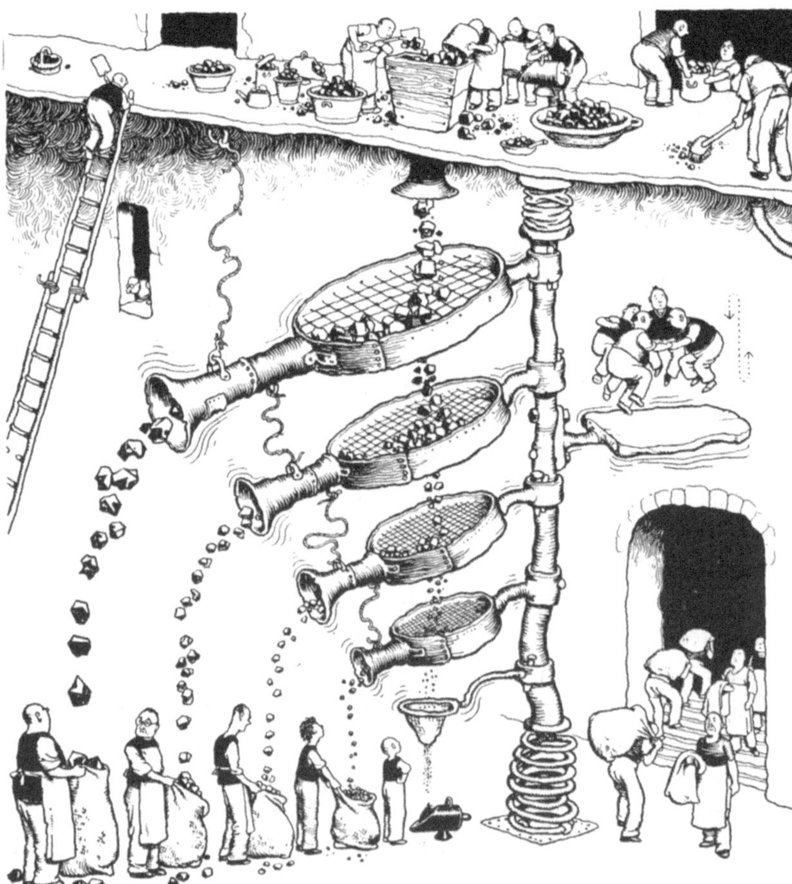

Coke Grading*

* Reproduced from *The Gentle Art of Advertising* by W. Heath Robinson, published by Gerald Duckworth & Co Ltd, London 1979, p. 88.

Contents

List of participants

Dr Adrian Barnes (A.B.)
Barnet General Hospital, Wellhouse Lane, Barnet EN5 3DJ, UK

Mr Peter Buchan (P.B.)
St James' University Hospital, Beckett Street, Leeds LS9 7TF, UK

Professor Shu Chien (S.C.)
Physiology Department, Columbia University College of Physicians and Surgeons, 630 S. 168th Street, New York, USA

Mr John Dormandy (J.D.)
St James' Hospital, Sarsfeld Road, London SW12 8HW, UK

Professor Albrecht Ehrly (A.E.)
Universitätskliniken, Frankfurt am Main 70, Federal Republic of Germany

Professor Sandro Forconi (S.F.)
Istituto di Patologia Speciale Medica, Universita di Siena, Istituti Clinici, Viale Bracci, 53100 Siena, Italy

Professor Peter Gaehtgens (P.G.)
Freie Universität Berlin, Arminallee 22, D-1000 Berlin 33

Professor Maxime Hanss (M.H.)
Université Paris Nord, UER Experimentale, 74 Rue Marcel Cachin, 9300 Bobigny, France

Dr Irene Juhan (I.J.)
Laboratoire Central d'Hématologie, Hôpital de la Timoni, 13385 Marseille

Professor Pierre Leblond (P.L.)
Department of Medicine, Hospital du Saint-Sacrement, 1050 Chemin Ste-Foy, Quebec G1S 4L8, Canada

Dr Gordon Lowe (G.L.)
Department of Medicine, Glasgow Royal Infirmary Glasgow G4 OSF, UK

Dr Georges Marcel (G.A.M.)
Laboratoires Hoechst, 3 Av. du General de Gaulle, 92800 Puteaux, France

Professor Herbert Meiselman (H.M.)
USC School of Medicine, 2025 Zonal Avenue (126 Mudd), Los Angeles, CA 90033, USA

Professor Holger Schmid-Schönbein (H.S-S.)
Abteilung Physiologie, Medizinische Fakultät, Rheinisch-Westfälische Technische Hochschule, Neuklinikum, Forckenbeckstrasse, Aachen, Federal Republic of Germany

Professor Richard Skalak (R.S.)
Bioengineering Institute, Columbia University, 610 Seeley W. Mudd Building, New York, NY 10027, USA

Professor Jean-Francois Stoltz (JF.S.)
Centre Regional de Transfusion Sanguine, Brabois 54500, Vandoeuvre-les-Nancy, France

Professor John Stuart (J.S.)
Department of Haematology, The Medical School, Vincent Drive, Birmingham B15 2TJ, UK

Professor Paul Teitel (P.T.)
Physiology Department, Rheinisch-Westfälische Technische Hochschule, Neuklinikum, Forckenbeckstrasse, Aachen, Federal Republic of Germany

Welcome

Sir John Stallworthy

It is my pleasure and privilege to welcome you back to the Royal Society of Medicine. We are particularly delighted to do this because it is not usual after a meeting as successful as you had last year to find that the productive work is still continuing and those responsible for the first meeting want to go on with working groups. It was a great pleasure to learn this is what you were doing when John spoke to us about this meeting and we were anxious to do anything we could to provide facilities for you. I hope you will not only enjoy this meeting but that you will find that it is even more productive than the main one last year, which we look back on as a memorable occasion. I think you will find the acoustics in this room are good. It is a Council room and we do not normally need microphones in the room at Council meetings, but all your proceedings as you know are being taped for sound and some of it also on videotape. I think you would feel it appropriate for me to pay a tribute from the Royal Society of Medicine, and on your behalf as well, to Hoechst, which has been most generous in giving a substantial donation with no strings attached to the Royal Society of Medicine and to John to make this meeting possible. I think there is no reference to them anywhere but it is a very generous thing to do and we are most grateful.

I am going to wish you well and declare the meeting open and ask Dr Georges Marcel if he would care to make his contribution. Then I will vacate this chair to Professor Gaehtgens. I wish you well.

Welcome

G.A. Marcel

Sir John, ladies and gentlemen. I am very happy to welcome you on behalf of the French Group on the Study of Red Cell Filtration. I have been trying to think of what filtration has to do with the countries present and of what links all these countries together. I think that as far as red cells are concerned, Great Britain has an eminent position thanks to William Hewson, who was the first to write that red cells are not always globular. I think that is one of our prime concerns. He had very modern thoughts because he also wrote that white cells were easily overlooked, which is another one of our acute problems. William Hewson went even further because he developed links with the United States at this early stage as he dedicated his most important book on the lymphatic system to Benjamin Franklin. But there are so many other reasons for our American friends to be here, especially their responsibility for so much of our knowledge in this field. Our friends from Germany are especially welcome. I must say that personally I am a fan of Sherlock Holmes. Yesterday I managed to find the original edition of 'His Last Bow' in Piccadilly and I am very excited and happy about that. Nevertheless what has all this to do with Sherlock Holmes? Well, we are near Baker Street which as you all know is the home of the great man. How is Germany linked to Holmes? The preferred hero of Paul Erlich was Sherlock Holmes, and how can we link Paul Erlich to all this? Well, Erlich was as you all well know staining cells and smears with dyes made by Hoechst and this allowed to distinguish structures between the different blood cells and again red cells and white cells. As far as Canada is concerned I think it is in Toronto that the oldest human red cells have been described. That is because they are very specialised in the study of mummies. It is in Toronto that the Egyptian mummy Nakt was dissected, studied and his red cells visualised by scanning electron microscope. Italy is the country of Bizzozego, linked to Germany because he studied with Virchow in Berlin. Bizzozego found that non-nucleated red cells came from nucleated red ones, which is of course crucial for us. Last of all France. Well, France is I should say last and alas because we have a lot of shame to recover from. When Bizzozego made his beautiful discovery Georges Hayem in France wrote an entire book to prove he was wrong, and that certainly red cells could not come from a nucleated precursor. So I think we still have a lot to do in France. Now, all that shows that nothing is simple and I think that is why we are all together, hopefully for success and clarity and for that anyhow I wish you all 'bonne chance'.

Introduction

Peter Gaehtgens

Sir John, ladies and gentlemen. I think we should start right away and I will just bother you with a few technical comments. As was already mentioned by Sir John, the entire meeting will be recorded on tape and immediately transcribed so as to make possible a publication in book form which will thus cover the entire discussion in addition to the presentations. Also your slides and transparencies will be copied immediately. The summarisers will then pre-edit all these transcripts and you will receive a copy. You thus have a chance to make alterations if necessary. The summarisers have been asked to critically sum up discussions and presentations and their impressions thereof, and this will then also be part of the publication.

The second point is that we have to think about the future. I would like to ask you to consider the following three or four points: The first question, of course, is what would be the appropriate time of the next meeting. I think we should make up our minds as to whether we should have this meeting at regular intervals, say, of one year or of two years. And we should also consider the question of whether future meetings should have the same format as the present one. The next point to be considered is the place of the next meeting: Would you prefer this working group to reconvene in London in this setting for instance at the Royal Society of Medicine which has been extremely rewarding in the past, or would you rather prefer the meeting to be held in another place, possibly in conjunction with any other scientific conference that you might want to attend. Finally, the question of whether or not the scope of the activities of this group should remain as it has been or whether it should be expanded. Would you prefer to cover other problems associated with what we could loosely call red cell deformability or should we stay within the framework of filtration as such? Towards the end of this meeting we can go through a short discussion of future plans. I hope that we can come up with some final conclusions as to how to proceed.

We should now start with the first session on ideal sampling techniques, the effects of anticoagulants, storage conditions and temperature of measurement. You will recall that this was a major point of the discussion last year and that some members of the group had at that time indicated their willingness to focus their interest and their activity on this problem. John Stuart was kind enough to compose this session and he will also start with the first presentation.

SESSION 1

Consideration of the ideal sampling technique, anticoagulant, storage conditions and temperature of measurement

J.S. During the 1981 meeting of the Working Group on Red Cell Deformability Professor Hanss, Dr Juhan and I were asked to look at the effect of different anticoagulants on blood samples taken for filtration studies. This proved more difficult than anticipated since, first of all, there were considerable technical differences in the filtration equipment in use in our three laboratories. The three of us therefore met in Paris to rationalise methodology and this is now almost complete. Some joint experiments have been possible during the rationalisation period and I shall present the results obtained by Dr Juhan and myself; Professor Hanss will then present the Paris data.

The second major difficulty was that a number of other factors, not only the anticoagulant, have the potential to influence the filtration of red cells if there is any delay between the time of venepuncture and the test. The blood sampling technique itself, as shown in Fig. 1.1, may be important. Clearly, for rheological studies on patients with diabetes mellitus, it is important to state whether the patient is fasting or has just eaten. The smoking history of the patient, including the time of the last cigarette, may also be important. For out-patients, it may be beneficial to provide a period of rest to minimise the effects of stress. Out-patients should also be studied at the same time of day unless circadian rhythm effects can be safely excluded.

The technique used to obtain a blood sample is, by analogy with blood taken for tests of a prothrombotic tendency, also of potential importance. Venous occlusion should be minimal, a small bore needle should be avoided, forceable suction should be avoided, and the first few millilitres of blood discarded. The nature of the container used (plastic or siliconized) should be stated and the storage conditions until the test is performed clearly defined. The last factor is so important, and has such a dominant effect on red cell filtration, that we cannot yet define the importance of the preceding factors listed until the effects of storage have been worked out.

The variables involved in blood storage are shown in Fig. 1.2. When whole blood is stored prior to testing, then the storage temperature (37° C, 4° C or ambient), the anticoagulant used (EDTA, heparin or citrate), the duration of

Blood sampling technique Variables	
Preparation of patient	Obtaining sample
Fasting or pre- / post-meal	Venous or arterial blood
Smoking	Tourniquet or not
Supine for 10–15 min	Needle size – 19 or 21 G
Circadian rhythm	Suction (syringe/vacutainer) or not
	Discard initial few ml
	Container – plastic/glass
	Storage conditions until test

Fig. 1.1

storage, and whether the blood remains static or agitated on a roller-mixer should all be carefully defined. More complex *in vitro* investigations (e.g. the effects of drugs on erythrocyte deformability) pose even greater technical problems requiring rigorous investigation of the effects of storage in buffer (as compared with plasma) with or without added albumin, fibrinogen, cholesterol and glucose. The effects of temperature on the rate of metabolic depletion during storage, Ca^{2+} chelation with EDTA (and to a lesser extent with citrate but not with heparin), ATP depletion with time, and the effects of continuous agitation are all of potential importance.

The first three variables in Fig. 1.2 (effect of temperature, anticoagulant and time delay) are probably the most important. Not only are their effects inter-related but also their effects differ according to the filtration method used. The original Birmingham positive-pressure filtration technique (Fig. 1.3; Kenny *et al.*, 1981, Clinical Hemorheology, *1*, 135–146) utilised washed erythrocytes re-

Blood storage conditions until test Variables	
Whole blood	Erythrocyte suspension
Temperature	In – Plasma
Anticoagulant – EDTA, heparin, citrate	Buffer ± albumin
Time delay	fibrinogen
Static or agitated	cholesterol
	glucose
	Temperature
	Anticoagulant – Ca^{2+} chelation
	Time delay – ATP depletion
	Static or agitated

Fig. 1.2

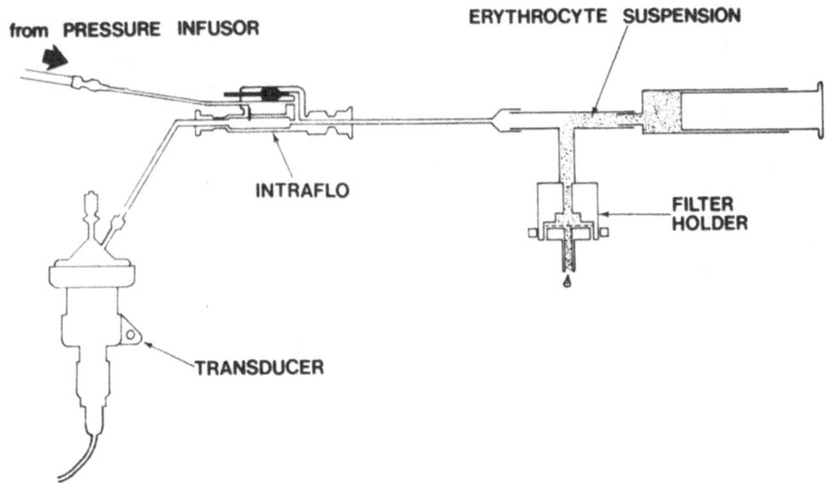

Fig. 1.3

suspended at a haematocrit of approximately 0.01 (1%) and filtered at room temperature. The filtrate was therefore free of contaminating plasma protein and contained very few platelets (approximately 0.5×10^9/l), but there were contaminating leucocytes. The method is currently being modified, by a pre-filtration step, to remove leucocytes but the data I shall present today were performed using the original technique. Our data and, I suspect, the data presented by all of us today, will therefore reflect the effect of temperature, anticoagulants, and time delay on leucocytes as well as on erythrocytes.

The first question, using this technique, concerns the effect of temperature during storage for up to 6 hours in K_2EDTA (Fig. 1.4). This figure shows the mean values for blood taken from 12 healthy individuals. The vertical axis represents the percentage change in red cell filtration ratio (pressure generated above the filter by the erythrocyte suspension compared with buffer alone) during 6 minutes' pumping time in relation to an initial value of 100%. The specimens stored at 4° C, but rewarmed to room temperature before filtering, showed a significant increase in red cell rigidity over the 6 hour period compared with no significant increase for specimens stored at 37° C or at room temperature. Wood and Beutler in 1967 (Journal of Laboratory and Clinical Medicine, *70*, 287–294) reported that the Na^+/K^+-ATPase in the red cell membrane was temperature sensitive and only 1/1000th as active at 4° C as at 37° C. Our samples stored at 4° C may therefore have shown cation changes. Dr Peter Weissberg (Department of Therapeutics and Clinical Pharmacology, University of Birmingham) has measured intracellular Na^+ and K^+ in these stored samples and

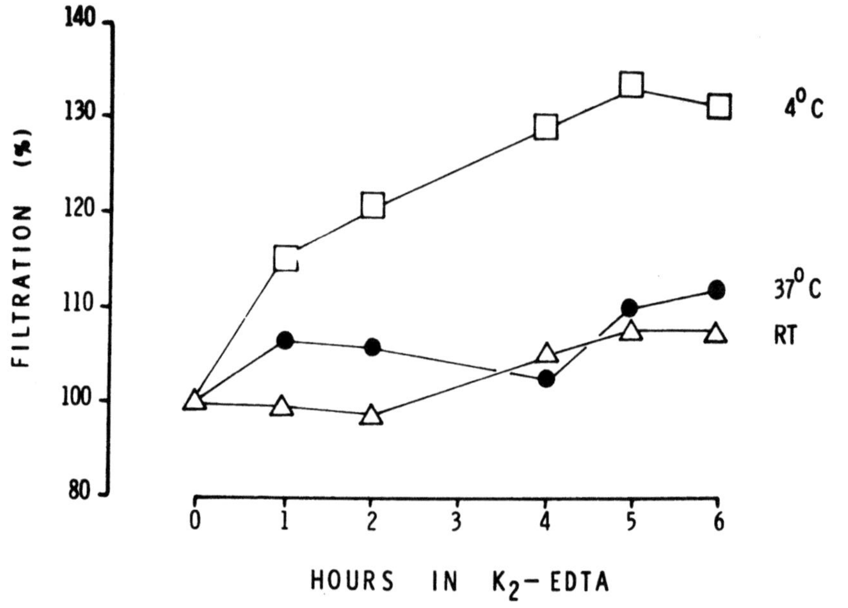

Fig. 1.4

shown that there is no significant change over 6 hours at room temperature for any of the three anticoagulants. Storage for 6 hours at 4° C, however, resulted in significant increases in intracellular Na^+ and an even greater decrease in intracellular K^+ for all three anticoagulants (pers. commun.). The net loss of intracellular cation may cause slight cell dehydration with a consequent loss of deformability.

The conclusion we have drawn from these results is that one should avoid storage at 4° C since erythrocyte cation changes occur, during 6 hours' storage, that may affect erythrocyte deformability. We do not know whether storage for a shorter period of time has a significant effect on cell cation content.

H.M. Are these changes reversible? Were the specimens rewarmed – it is normally expected that one rewarms whole blood to counter the effects you have described.

J.S. We have not yet looked at reversibility. The cells stored at 4° C were rewarmed to room temperature before filtering. The cation measurements were, however, performed at 4° C.

The next stage was to ask which of the three anticoagulants (EDTA, heparin or citrate) we should use when blood is stored at room temperature prior to storage. The only previous data I am aware of are those of Schröer and colleagues. (IVème Séminaire du Groupe de Travail sur la Filtration Érythrocytaire, La Baule 1979). These workers used a whole-blood filtration method and found a significantly slower filtration rate with heparin, and also citrate, compared with EDTA. When the buffy coat was removed, and the red cells washed before filtering at a haematocrit of 0.40 (40%), there was no longer any difference between the three anticoagulants. Furthermore, scanning electron photomicrographs of the Nuclepore filter surface showed pore plugging with platelets after filtration of whole blood taken into heparin or citrate. This was not seen when EDTA was the anticoagulant.

Since the Birmingham technique employs a virtually platelet-free filtrate we thought that we should repeat these studies. Figure 1.5 shows the mean values for the red cell filtration ratio (again converted to percentage change in the vertical axis) for blood taken from 12 healthy individuals into CPD-A_1 (citrate-phosphate-dextrose-adenine as used for Blood Bank storage prior to transfusion), sodium citrate (0.105 M), lithium heparin, and K_2EDTA. As before, the anticoagulated samples were stored for 6 hours at room temperature. Each of the anticoagulants, with the exception of K_2EDTA, caused a progressive and significant increase in filtration ratio (pressure above the filter) with time. Since our filtrate contained some contaminating leucocytes and since we used a long filtration time (6 minutes) our results may again reflect an artefact – that is, an effect of heparin and citrate causing leucocyte aggregation or plugging of the filter. We therefore plan to repeat these experiments using a leucocyte-free filtrate.

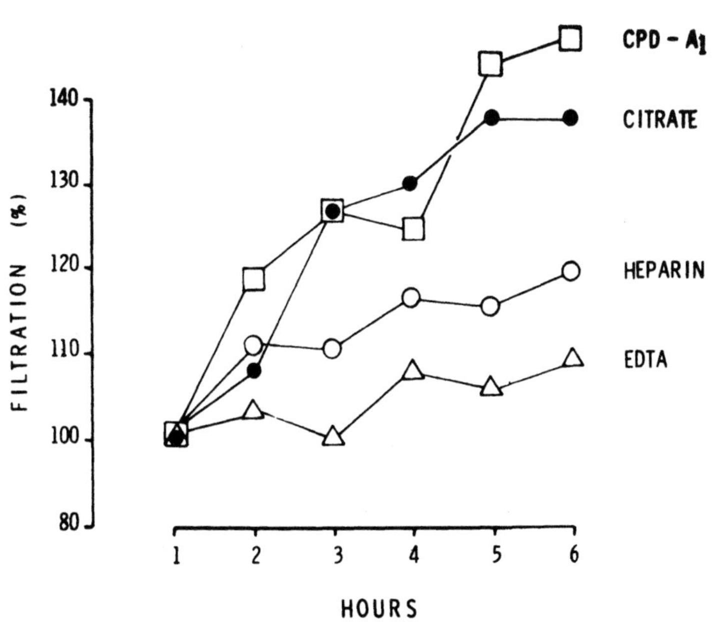

Fig. 1.5

An alternative approach to avoiding the effect of contaminating leucocytes, is to use a method that is insensitive to leucocyte plugging of the filter. The Hanss Hémorhéomètre (Fig. 1.6; Hanss, M., Biorheology, *20*, 199–211, 1983) may be one such method since only the first 0.5–2.0 seconds of filtration time are measured. When we used this instrument, the results (Fig. 1.7) showed no significant change in filtration time (again converted to percentage change on the vertical axis) with any of the three anticoagulants over a storage time of 6 hours at room temperature.

Finally, we have not found, during the 6 hour storage period, any major difference between the three anticoagulants for pH, red cell size (using the Coulter Channelyzer), or osmolality. There is, however, evidence that all three anticoagulants result in some erythrocyte (or leucocyte) damage during storage since the plasma LDH (lactate dehydrogenase) level, as shown in Fig. 1.8, increases progressively with time over 6 hours. The vertical axis shows both the percentage change and the original LDH values in units per litre. The increase in LDH over 6 hours is statistically significant ($P<0.01$) for all three anticoagulants so this cannot be the explanation for the difference between EDTA and heparin/citrate in the filterability studies.

In conclusion, Mr Chairman, these preliminary and unpublished data from Dr Juhan and me suggest that blood samples should not be stored at 4°C prior to erythrocyte filtration studies (since cation changes may occur) and that EDTA is

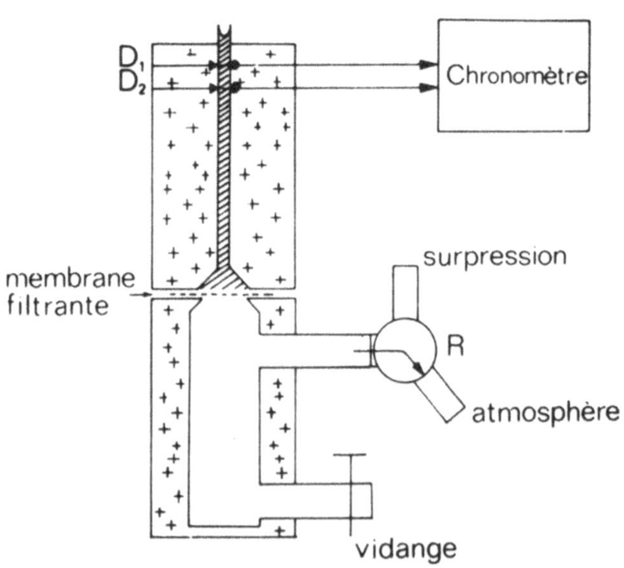

Fig. 1.6

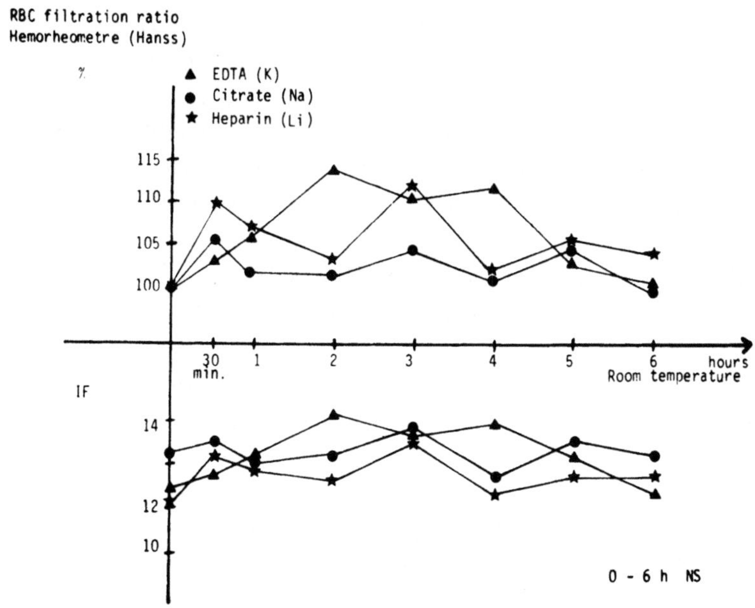
RBC filtration ratio
Hemorheometre (Hanss)
%
EDTA (K)
Citrate (Na)
Heparin (Li)
115
110
105
100
30 min.
1
2
3
4
5
6
hours
Room temperature
IF
14
12
10
0 - 6 h NS

Fig. 1.7

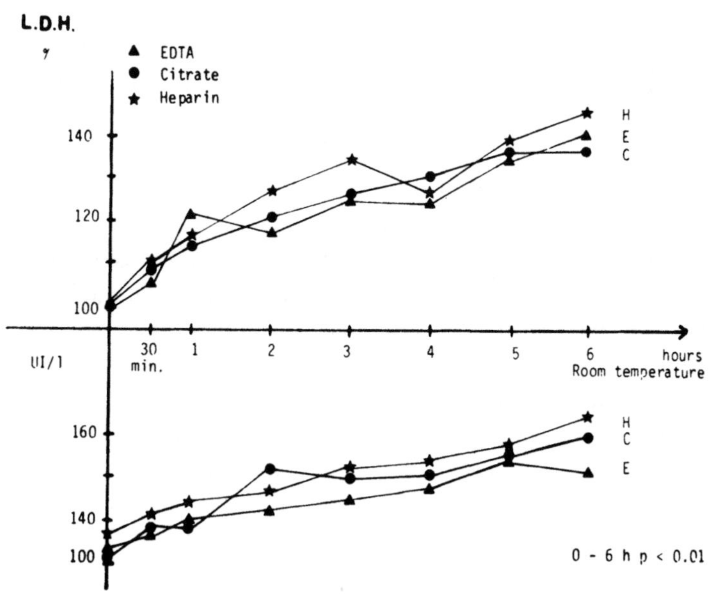
L.D.H.
%
EDTA
Citrate
Heparin
140
120
100
H
E
C
30 min.
1
2
3
4
5
6
hours
Room temperature
UI/1
160
140
100
H
C
E
0 - 6 h p < 0.01

Fig. 1.8

the anticoagulant of choice (to avoid platelet aggregation and pore blockage) if a whole-blood filtration system is used. Furthermore, since washed erythrocyte suspensions may contain a variable proportion of leucocytes, EDTA should again be used (to avoid probable effects of heparin/citrate on leucocytes with consequential pore blockage). There are no data yet available on the effects of anticoagulants on leucocyte-free suspensions of erythrocytes.

P.G. We should now open this up for a short discussion before we move to the next presentation.

M.H. All the figures given were for washed cells?

J.S. Yes, the cells were washed three times in phosphate-buffered saline to remove plasma protein.

H.M. I've been trying to do a quick calculation to relate the loss of intracellular potassium, and gain of intracellular sodium, with the lack of any measurable change in osmolality of the external medium. It looks like you have a net loss from the cell to the extracellular medium of about 20 mmols per kg of dry weight red cell mass. This should have given you some change in the osmolality of the external medium unless when you brought the cells back up to room temperature, the cation changes were restored to normal.

J.S. Your point about rewarming is very important and clearly the cation changes should be studied over a much shorter timescale than 6 hours and we should also see what the effects of rewarming are.

P.B. In your slide on the sampling conditions you mentioned circadian variation. I would, as a gynaecologist, put in a plug for menstrual variation because it's been shown that there is quite a change in erythrocyte deformability as measured by filtration in the premenstrual phase of the cycle. Ladies become more tense perhaps, but their red cells become more flexible, at that time. Perhaps that is something to be thought about in filtration studies on women.

J.D. Did you say that there was no significant change in the stored blood over 6 hours in pH and is that not surprising?

J.S. Yes, perhaps, but there was no major change.

P.L. The question of the use of Vacutainers for taking blood samples for filtration studies is important. We use Vacutainers all the time and have not seen, in comparative studies, much of a difference in the results of our tests. I don't know about the experience of other people around the table.

S.C. We have not done any systematic evaluation of this problem but we have not seen any demonstrable effect due to the vacuum technique.

J.S. I don't think there are any hard data on that. Dr Leblond wrote to me about this point and we have started a comparative study. So far (13 paired samples), we have not found a significant difference between a conventional venepuncture and a Vacutainer sample.

P.G. Can I ask a simple question, John. You have given mean values on all of your slides in order to appreciate the changes that you have seen as a function of time, or temperature, or anticoagulant. What is the variability of an individual measurement; what is the spread of the data within each group?

J.S. The data given were the means for 12 specimens from normal people. We did not assume that the data were normally distributed so the analyses were done using either a Mann-Whitney U test or a Wilcoxon paired test and significance was based on that. The coefficient of variation of the technique is under 10% for replicate specimens.

S.C. John, you showed very clearly that 4° C storage is not desirable. These tests were done in a suspension containing a significant amount of white cells. Did you repeat the temperature experiment with a reduced white cell concentration and did you try it with Professor Hanss' Hémorhéomètre?

J.S. No, we haven't done temperature studies with the Hémorhéomètre and we have yet to repeat the Birmingham study of different temperatures and different anticoagulants using a leucocyte-free technique.

S.C. My question is really whether the 4° C effect is mediated through the leucocytes rather than the red cells.

J.S. Yes, and I think everything I have said, and everything that will be said in this session, might equally apply to leucocytes rather than erythrocytes.

P.G. Thank you very much John Stuart. Let's move on to the next contribution then, by Professor Hanss.

M.H. Well, I will first speak about anticoagulants. We have made many measurements with our apparatus, about 2000 different samples, and we have found a significant increase in our filtration index (indicating loss of deformability) when the samples were taken into EDTA as compared with heparin. We therefore thought that heparin was a better anticoagulant because the red cells were more pliable than with EDTA, but this is not a logical reason. I mean the choice of an anticoagulant is a matter of philosophy, or what you are looking for, so I will present one slide which gives some results obtained on diabetic patients (Fig. 1.9). It shows that if you make the measurement on heparin samples then you get a very significant difference between diabetic patients and

		Diabetics	Controls	p
F. (Hep)	N:	311 (76)	77	<0.001
	<IF>:	11.44 (11.30)	9.97	
	σ:	2.82 (3.01)	2.47	
F. (EDTA)	N:	293 (53)	30	N.S.
	<IF>:	15.01 (14.4)	13.06	
	σ:	6.68 (3.06)	2.52	

Fig. 1.9 Values in brackets refer to a previous independent study.

controls, if you study a big population, but if you use EDTA then you don't get any significant difference. So, if you want to show that red blood cells from diabetic patients are less pliable, then you use heparin. And if you want to show that there is no difference then you use EDTA. Also, I think heparin is better because the SD is much lower than for EDTA samples and that is the reason for the non-significance with EDTA.

We have also found that the storage condition and the delay between the suspension preparation and measurement is important but we apparently did not get the same results as Stuart. This may be because we always use Vacutainer samples and test the specimens in the Hémorhéomètre. We don't find any difference in filtration rate using the Hémorhéomètre when the blood sample is left at room temperature, say for one hour roughly. It doesn't change. However, when you keep it longer, say for 3 or 4 hours, in that case it starts changing. If the same sample is put at 4° C then it doesn't change at all. So we don't find any filtration rate differences between stored blood samples at 4° C and measurement made, say, in just the half hour after the venepuncture. Any delay after preparation of the red cell suspension and the measurement is more important and we have observed an increase, which can go as high as 50–60% in our filtration index, when you put the red cell in the buffer for one hour. So the proposition is to measure the filtration rate as soon as possible once you have prepared the erythrocyte suspension in buffer.

Now about the temperature effect proper on the filtration index, that is, on the red blood cell rheology. If one uses a simple method where the result is given as time flow, then the temperature effects are very high because viscosity is highly temperature dependent. But if you use a method where a ratio of erythrocyte suspension to buffer is measured, the temperature effect is damped. But in that case, a temperature effect remains because the temperature coefficients of the viscosity of the buffers and the temperature coefficient of the rheological properties of the red blood cells are different. This temperature effect on the filtration index is shown in Fig. 1.10. We have measured at 25° C as our reference level. The temperature was then lowered or increased and we measured the new filtration index. Of course when we have a very high temperature (above 45° C) then the filtration index (which is higher when the cell is stiffer) gets very high indeed since this is the well-known spectrin denaturation effect. If the temperature changes by, say, 5° C around 25° C, which is quite often observed in laboratories, then you have 5–10% difference in the filtration index. So if the temperature is not controlled there can be about 10% fluctuation. Therefore our conclusion is that we have to control the temperature if we want to have precise measurements.

P.G. Thank you very much Professor Hanss. Now Pierre Leblond wants to comment.

P.L. I just want to come back to Professor Hanss about the storage time of red cells suspended in buffer compared with whole blood. We have observed that the

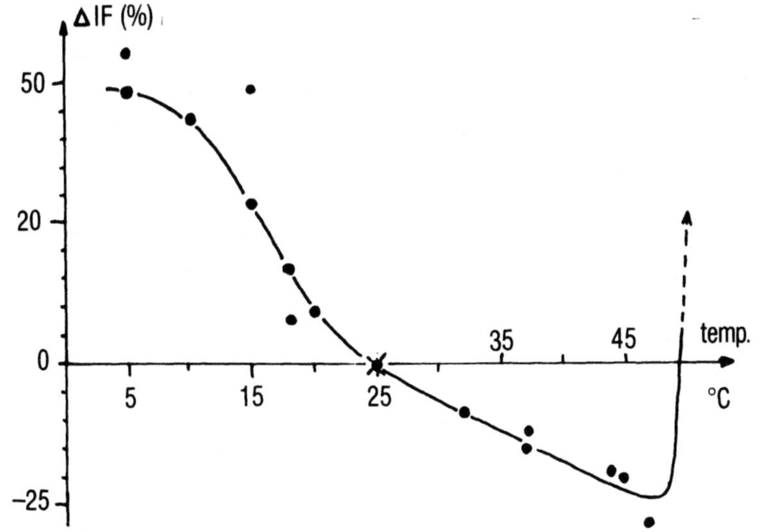

Fig. 1.10

haematocrit of the suspension is important and if you go to 0.01 (1%) haematocrit and below you can afford only a very short delay before testing. You have to be very quick, otherwise there is a change in cell volume and we have observed this in our experiments. We usually test within 5 minutes. I think it is an important point and the lower the cell concentration the faster you must act. Would you agree with this?

S.F. I completely agree with this. When we take a red cell and wash and brush and shave that cell we no longer have that same red cell after one hour but something quite different. But if we study red cells immediately after venepuncture we have a more physiological index of these phenomena. This is important for clinical work.

I.J. An important point is that you have calcium in your buffer and, in your technique, the EDTA-anticoagulated blood is not washed so you have a little plasma left.

M.H. A very small amount – about 1 part in 1,000.

I.J. We have seen a little coagulation in EDTA blood when a buffer containing calcium is added.

M.H. This is why EDTA-anticoagulated samples are less reproducible than heparin.

A.E. Coming back to Pierre Leblond's point, I am sure he is right but if you dilute your blood with plasma we have never seen the changes he described.

P.L. I agree. I was talking about non-protein media (i.e. a buffer solution). If you go below 0.01 (1%) haematocrit you'd better act fast because something is going to happen.

H.M. I am interested in the temperature effect. We know that the viscosity of the membrane is exquisitely sensitive to temperature whereas the shear modulus is not, so that your increase in filtration index with lower temperature could reflect the membrane viscosity getting higher with lower temperature.

M.H. In addition, there are quite a number of studies on the effect of temperature on the microviscosity of membrane lipid.

H.M. How do we relate this to the observations pointed out earlier about loss of intracellular potassium and cell dehydration. Is that part of what's happening at the lower temperatures do you think?

M.H. I don't know but it happens also to red cell ghosts.

S.C. With reference to what Dr Meiselman just asked about the membrane viscosity, we have used the micropipette technique to measure the viscosity of the membrane during deformation and during recovery as a function of temperature. There was an inverse relationship as you have shown for the filtration test so the same thing happens and, interestingly enough, we also found a transition temperature at around 18–20° C.

I would also like to ask a question about the effect of temperature. I think Professor Stuart said it is better to store at room temperature and here you say it is better to store at 4° C. I think maybe one of the differences is the way the sample is stored. Maybe with whole blood, with the white cells present, it is better to store at room temperature. Once you wash the red cell you should not store it, as you pointed out Professor Hanss, but if you do want to store it, it is maybe better to store at 4° C? I am just venturing this as a way of reconciling the apparent differences and I wonder whether you have any thoughts about this.

M.H. I was talking about whole blood at 4° C so I don't know the answer to your question.

J.D. Professor Chien just asked the question I was going to ask, but we did do some experiments on temperature and storage and 4° C does seem to be worse than at room temperature for storing whole blood.

M.H. Measurements being made on whole blood or a cell suspension?

J.D. Both.

J.S. The difference may be that Professor Hanss' technique is largely insensitive to white cell effects. This may explain the difference between the Birmingham filtration method which is sensitive to white cell changes, whereas Professor Hanss' very short filtration time is probably insensitive to what happens to white cells. Hence he finds a different result a 4° C than we do.

P.G. Thank you very much Professor Hanss. The next speaker will be Mr Peter Buchan, again on temperature and time delay.

P.B. When I started my filtration studies using the method of Reid *et al.*, 1976 (Journal of Clinical Pathology, *29*, 855–858) – that is, using a whole blood suspension and measuring erythrocyte deformability by filtration through a

5 μm pore-size filter – I found quite a significant drop off in filtration rate with fall in temperature even in the range of temperature in my laboratory during summer–winter. As part of my study I was particularly interested in the effects of plasma viscosity, because I was viewing a group of patients with very widely varying plasma viscosities, and so the obvious experiment was to look at the effects of temperature on plasma viscosity. Using a suspension of erythrocytes in their own plasma, with a haematocrit of about 0.30 (30%), I found that the erythrocyte filtration rate fell off with a decrease in temperature (Fig. 1.11), but when I measured the plasma viscosity of each of these samples I found that the plasma viscosity was particularly sensitive to changes in temperature (Fig. 1.12). As a result, when I corrected my erythrocyte filtration rate for the plasma viscosity I found no, or very little, change with temperature. So my conclusion from this was that I was seeing a plasma viscosity effect in the system that I was

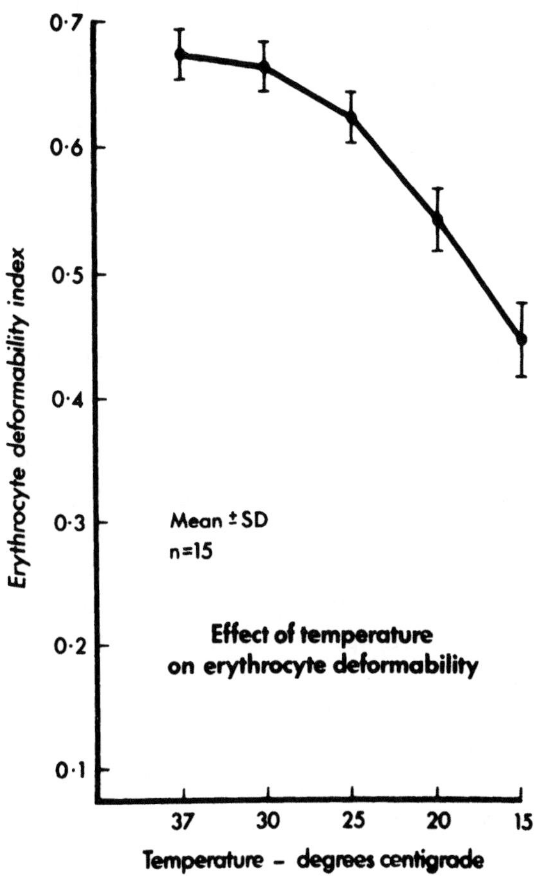

Fig. 1.11

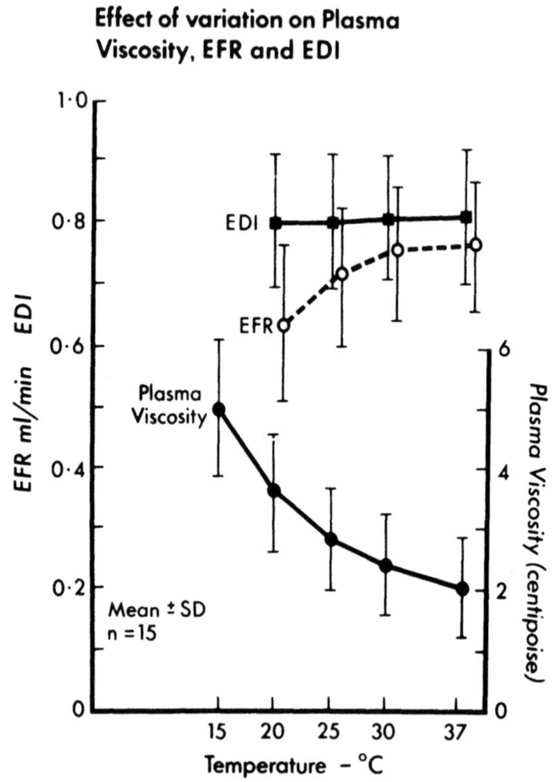

Fig. 1.12

using. My last point concerns delay in measurement. I found that, with storage at 37° C, for up to 6 hours, there was a marked fall off in erythrocyte deformability after 2 hours. So for my experiment the critical time for measurement, which would seem to be in agreement with the last speaker, is about 2 hours from venepuncture; thereafter I found, in EDTA samples stored at 37° C, a fairly rapid fall off in deformability.

A.B. Last year we presented similar data, using the same method, and found the effect of small temperature changes at 25° C to be minimal but at 4° C and 37° C the cells were a lot more temperature sensitive, or the system was a lot more temperature sensitive.

P.B. I didn't look at the extremes but studied only the range from 15 to 37° C.

H.M. Isn't there now a dichotomy between this and Professor Hanss' presentation in the effect of temperature on filtration? What is the difference?

M.H. The difference is in the vertical axis – what is measured – that is all. I feel that you have to use a method which is sensitive to the individual red blood cell, if this is the problem you are interested in, and not to the interaction between cells caused by plasma.

J.D. Our results are similar in that we find an effect of temperature on whole blood filtration but if you correct for the change in viscosity of the plasma, or express the result as a ratio, then almost all of the temperature effect is abolished, which I think is very much what the previous speakers have said.

H.S-S. We find that, in plasma, there is a temperature sensitivity in the sense that the relative flow rate decreases (by about 20–30%) with decrease in temperature. But results with the single cell rigidometer do not seem to be affected by temperature when we use washed cells. In other words, I am afraid that in all the whole blood filtration tests there is rouleaux formation induced by plasma factors with a very high temperature sensitivity of the adhesive forces and therefore of the probability of disrupting rouleaux.

P.G. Dr Forconi is next on the list of speakers and he will again talk about storage and temperature.

S.F. The purpose of our study was to control the influence of temperature on red cell filterability. We made a single modification to the original method of Reid *et al.* (1976) in order to keep the temperature constant during blood filtration. This modification consists of a temperature-controlled water jacket. We have used EDTA-anticoagulated whole blood from healthy donors and stored it in three different water baths at temperatures of 25°, 30° or 37° C respectively. To minimise the influence of the unavoidable delay between measurements, the order of the tests was changed during each experiment (Fig. 1.13). The time required for all the 15 tests for each donor was approximately 60 minutes. In each test, the volume of red blood cells (Vrbc) was calculated by dividing 60 by the time during which 1 ml of blood was filtered and multiplying it by the haematocrit. Then we calculated the mean value for each group of 5 tests and, successively, the mean value for those obtained in 6 donors. The higher the temperature the higher the filterability of the red cell proved to be (Fig. 1.14). In every group of 5 measurements we calculated also the relative standard de-

Study of the effect of temperature on red cell filterability

6 healthy voluntary donors
30 ml of whole blood + 0.6 ml of EDTA 10%
3 tubes 10 ml each
3 different water baths (25° = A; 30° = B; 37° = C)
5 tests for each tube changing the order for each donor
1) = A–B–C; 2) = B–C–A; 3) = C–A–B; 4) = A–B–C; 5) = B–C–A; 6) = C–A–B

$$V_{RBC} = 60/T \times HTC/100$$

Mean ± SD of each group of 5 V_{RBC} for each donor
Mean ± SD of 6 means at the same temperature
Relative standard deviation + 100 × SD/mean
Mean of the RSD at the same temperature

Fig. 1.13

Effect of temperature on red cell filterability
mean ± s.d.; n = 6

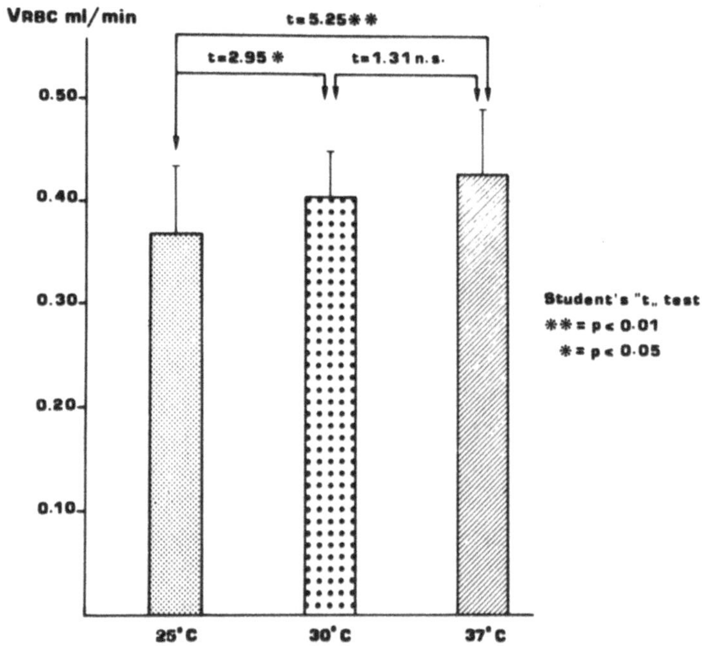

Fig. 1.14

viation. The mean value of the 6 relative standard deviations is shown in Fig. 1.15, the best relative standard deviation, which is 4%, being obtained at 37° C.

The conclusion from this first part of the study was that temperature changed the red cell filtration and that the method was much more reliable at 37° C. This finding reinforced our idea that we should not take measurements at room temperature but choose the same temperature in all parts of the world. Also, if we want to reproduce *in vitro* the passage of blood through the capillaries the least we can do is not change the temperature. Moreover, at 37° C the results are more reliable.

The second important problem that we have in red cell filtration is the storage of blood. Are we to measure immediately after venepuncture or can we wait? In order to study this we took blood from 6 healthy donors. Eighty milliliters of blood, anticoagulated in EDTA, were collected in 13 tubes (Fig. 1.16). The blood contained in the first tube was used immediately for red cell filtration, 4 tubes were stored at 37° C, 4 tubes at 25° C, and 4 tubes at 4° C. The measurements were taken after 30, 60, 120 and 180 minutes. The temperature of the filtration equipment was always 37° C and the operator was always the same. Also in this

Red cell filterability. Effect of temperature on the method
mean ± s.d.; n = 6

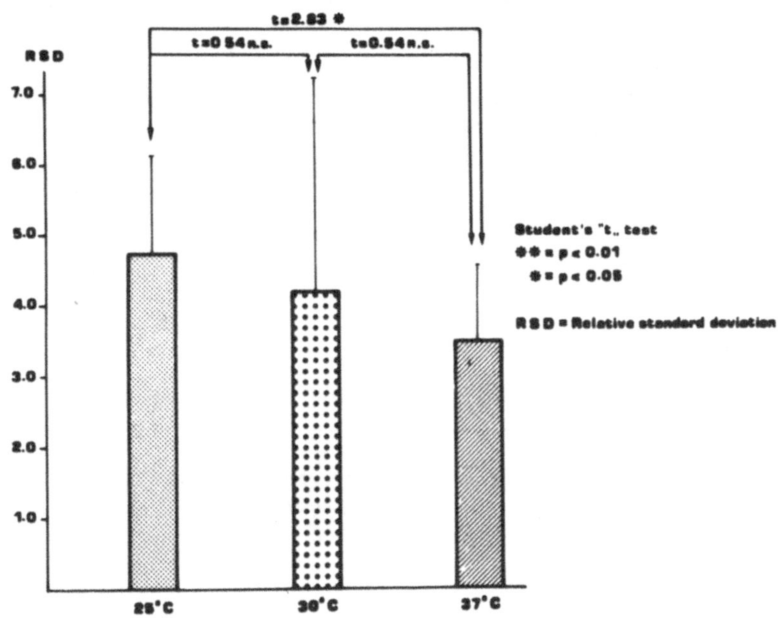

Fig. 1.15

case, in order to minimise the influence of the slight delay due to the order of the tests, the order was changed for each donor and the measurements for each different temperature started either 5 minutes before, or at the exact time, or 5 minutes after the expected time of storage.

From the results (Fig. 1.17) we can see there are no differences, and this is different from what I said last year, in the storage at 25° C and at 37° C but, in the blood stored at 4° C, we observed a surprising decrease in filtration time and an increase in Vrbc.

We tried to express these results using a mathematical function. This was not possible for blood stored at 4° C, while for 25° C and 37° C (Fig. 1.18) it was very easy to build a linear function of the decay of the values. This shows the relative decay every 5 minutes. After 5 minutes at 37° C, there is a fall of 2%, after 10 minutes of 3%, and so on and the results are quite similar for 37° and 25° C. These results confirm the important influence of the time of storage on filterability performed on whole blood. The reason for this behaviour is not completely clear.

In a pilot study, we studied also the pH and lactic acid concentration in the samples during storage at the various temperatures. The level of lactic acid was

Study of the effect of temperature on the storage of blood for red cell filterability

6 healthy voluntary donors
80 ml of whole blood + 1.6 ml of EDTA 10%
13 tubes 6 ml each
All measurements performed at 37° C
3 tests for each tube
1 tube immediately tested, 4 tubes stored at 37° C
4 tubes stored at 25° C, 4 tubes stored at 4° C
Tests performed after 30, 60, 120 and 180 minutes of storage

Fig. 1.16

Effect of storage temperature on red cell filterability
1 way an. o. va.; mean ± s.d.; n = 6

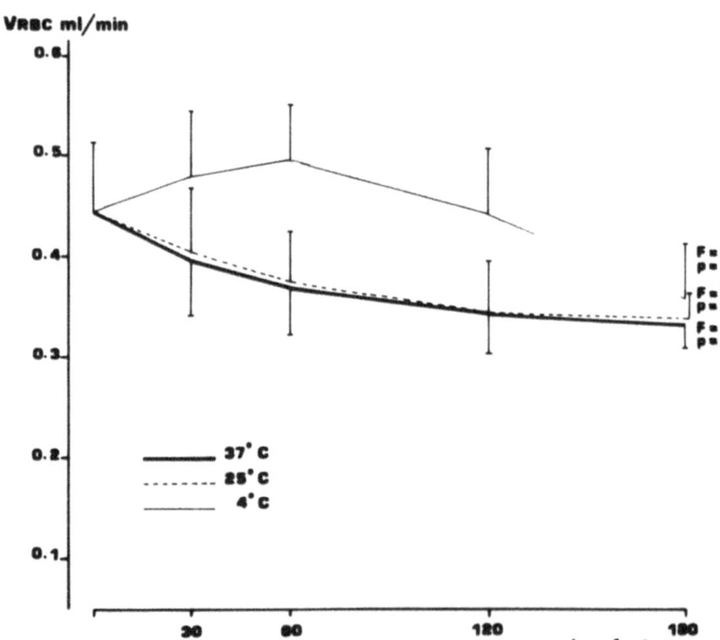

Fig. 1.17

Linear regression of red cell filterability during storage

				Y = AX + B				
Y = log % of decrease				X = time of storage				
37° C	A = −0.0013			B = 1.1997			R = 0.9910	
X =	0	5	10	15	20	25	30	60
% =	100	97.9	96.5	95.1	93.7	92.4	91.1	83.5
25° C	A = −0.0012			B = 1.998			R = 0.9979	
X =	0	5	10	15	20	25	30	60
% =	100	98.3	97.0	95.6	94.4	93.1	91.8	84.6

Fig. 1.18

clearly temperature dependent, and an increase in this metabolic product might be correlated with the decrease of deformability at either temperature. However, the increase in lactic acid is not synonymous with acidosis because, by measuring also the pH under the same conditions, we are not able to detect a significant change. There was a general tendency, but no more than a tendency, to a pH increase, probably due to loss of CO_2 from the samples.

Our findings suggest that it is not possible to store blood samples for red cell filterability at any optimal temperature, since, whether at room temperature or at 37° C or at 4° C, there are always important changes beginning in the first 10 minutes. In our studies we therefore always measure red cell filterability immediately after withdrawal.

P.G. Questions, comments?

P.T. I would like to make a single comment regarding nomenclature. Data have been presented here as red cell filterability while I gather from your presentation that you have worked with whole blood. So I think in order to avoid any possible confusion it would perhaps be preferable to express results in terms of whole blood filtration instead of red cell filtration because otherwise one cannot find out whether effects are to be related directly only to red cells or maybe to some other factors present in the blood which has been stored under your conditions.

S.F. Yes, I completely agree and if we want to relate filterability to the passage of whole blood through the capillaries then we should measure whole blood filterability.

H.M. I would like to return to this question of the inactivation at 4° C of the Na^+/K^+-ATPase. Your data showed that, with storage at 4° C, there is actually an initial increase in the flow followed by a drop back to the control value. It is interesting that, if you slightly dehydrate cells, just a little bit, you actually get a slight increase in 'deformability' even though you would argue that the internal viscosity went up a little. It turns out that the surface-to-volume ratio goes up more, and initially you get an increase in deformability, whatever that word means. So I think it is probably important to look at the time course of cell dehydration at 4° C and the time course of reversal when rewarming it to 25° or 37° C. Could any of this be a cell volume change consequent upon cooling to 4° C?

A.B. I also wondered if you had any data on pH in any of these experiments?

S.F. The general tendency is to a loss of CO_2 since we perform our measurements in open tubes and there is a tendency to alkalosis; but I think only a tendency because the results are not significant from the statistical point of view till the third hour. The lactic acid concentration also changed significantly but this is not synonymous with acidosis because in blood there is a compensation.

J.D. You showed results obtained at 10 minutes after withdrawing the blood and found that it makes a difference whether you measure 10 minutes or an hour later. I think all the previous presenters started measuring at one hour or at least their graphs started at about one hour. Am I right in thinking that you might all have missed an earlier change – in particular, John Stuart? Can he comment on what happens in the first 10 minutes?

J.S. The only experiment we have performed at 15 minutes from venepuncture showed no difference from the value obtained at 1 hour for blood taken into EDTA and stored at room temperature.

H.S-S. It is at least debatable whether the effects of temperature are intracellular or whether they are related to some other artefact which has a different temperature coefficient such as red cell aggregation, or a white cell or platelet effect. Platelets are extremely sensitive to hypothermia; this is a very important non-specific stimulus. Cooling at 4° C, and subsequent warming, is one of the best ways to activate platelets. So, while it is important to look at subtle changes in the MCV and surface area-to-volume ratio, I think we have no firm evidence that there really is a time-dependent change or a temperature-dependent change at the molecular or cellular level.

P.G. The next presentation will be given by Holger Schmid-Schönbein and will also deal with the effect of anticoagulants.

H.S-S. I have a terrible history of confusing matters but this has always been done inadvertently in the past. This time I do it on purpose! Professor Hanss was kind enough to give us one of his Hémorhéomètres and he told us that EDTA is not a good anticoagulant. Now, historically, when Volger and I started to use our filtration methods we came up with the recommendation to use EDTA at 1.5 mg per ml. The decision was based on the calculation of the coefficients of variation and on the time effects. When we used the heparin then available we found that, during storage for the first four hours, there was a significant drop in filtration but, more importantly, there was a significant increase in the coefficient of variation.

Now during this year, and of course after the meeting here in London in 1981, we looked back at this topic and it was Dr M. Singh with us who did most of the work; part of it was published as an abstract to the recent Jerusalem meeting. We have used four different methods (Fig. 1.19) – first is the polymicroviscometer (PMV), that is another way of describing Paul Teitel's paper-filter method, which is now automated (Filtrometer), and he has chosen to quantify the results in half filtration time. Then we have the Reid and Dormandy method (we use an 0.45 (45%)) haematocrit in saline; white cells and platelets being removed by removing the buffy coat). We then have the Hanss Hémorhéomètre (HR) filtration index and the single erythrocyte rigidometer (SER). With the latter we have the mean passage time in ms. It was Singh's idea to look at some subpopulations of cells that are very fast (i.e. under the conditions that he used they passed within 10–20 ms) and then cells which passed slowly (i.e. between 30–40 ms). At 41° C, we are already beginning to see a very significant increase in the mean passage time with a decrease in the fast population and an increase in the slow population so that the whole population is shifted.

Now using these four different techniques we also looked at the following anticoagulants – EDTA 1.5 mg/ml; heparin (Roche) and this is now a new chromatographed product; sodium citrate (3.5%) at a dilution of 1/10; and then acid-citrate-dextrose (ACD) as it is in the Travenol blood transfusion bag.

One of the things we found, as we looked into the distribution of the passage

	Temperatures			
	20° C	30° C	37° C	41° C
PMV				
Half filtration time (min)	12.1 ± 1.91^a	10.16 ± 1.64^b	11.5 ± 3.70	9.98 ± 2.95^a
R-D				
Flow rate (ml/min)	0.86 ± 0.21^a	0.83 ± 0.31^a	0.91 ± 0.36	0.78 ± 0.22^b
HR				
Filtration index	14.1 ± 4.03^a	12.3 ± 2.33^a	13.1 ± 2.72	11.2 ± 2.06^c
SER				
Erythrocytes % in 10–20 ms	52.7 ± 12.7^a	50.0 ± 13.4^a	52.4 ± 14.5	35.7 ± 16.5^d
Erythrocytes % in 30–40 ms	8.60 ± 2.50^a	7.42 ± 5.60^a	9.25 ± 6.50	16.0 ± 9.70^c
Mean passage time (ms)	27.2 ± 9.1^a	30.9 ± 10.4^a	30.8 ± 9.10	39.8 ± 9.90^d

^{a} NS, ^{b} $p<0.15$, ^{c} $p<0.05$, ^{d} $p<0.025$

A comparative analysis of the data shows that the temperature influences the flow behaviour of the erythrocytes through micropores to various extents in different techniques.

Fig. 1.19

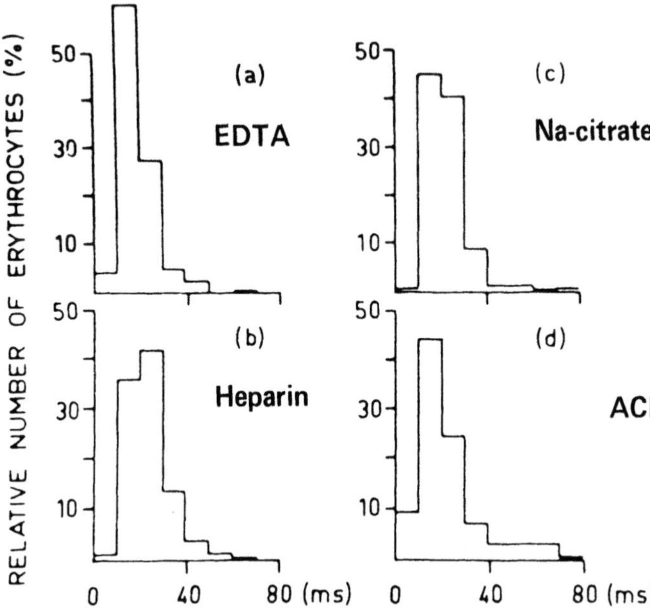

Fig. 1.20

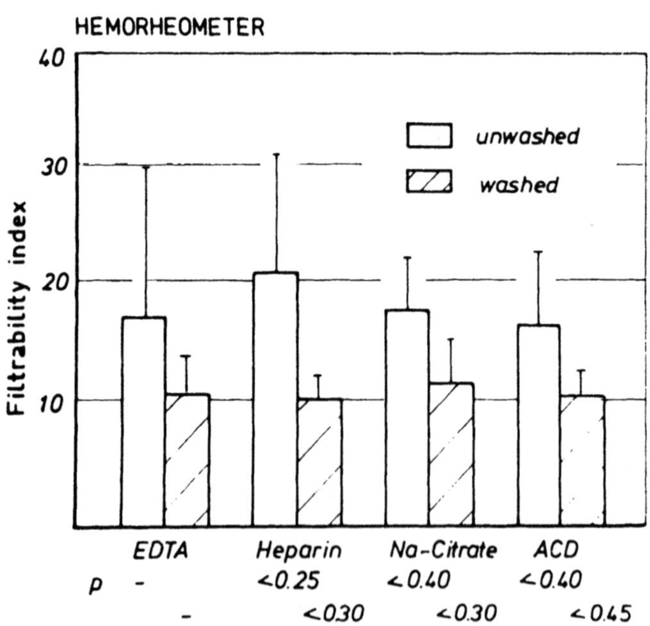

Fig. 1.21

time in the single erythrocyte rigidometer (Fig. 1.20), was that the slow population of red cells was very strongly affected by the use of the anticoagulant and it tended to disappear when we used EDTA. We then used the Hanss Hémorhéomètre and you can see (Fig. 1.21) that, in the washed samples, there is virtually no effect but if we used unwashed cells there was an effect. You can also see, and this is important, that with EDTA and heparin there is a surprising scatter and we are at a loss to explain this, why it is less in sodium citrate and ACD. With the Teitel Filtrometer (Fig. 1.22), which is essentially a micropolyviscometry of densely packed cells under very low shear stresses, washing has an enormous effect. In other words, washing the cells three times in buffered saline containing 0.25% human serum albumin produces a very significant effect. Over and above that, we can very clearly see that EDTA has by far the shortest half time, in other words the best flow. Much to our confusion, sodium citrate and ACD were exactly the opposite. Now mind you, in this system, the cell–cell interaction, as well as subtle details of the cytoplasmic viscosity and the viscous properties of the membrane, dominate the flow process in contrast to the other systems. Next, the Reid/Dormandy method (Fig. 1.23) shows the highest flow rate for EDTA and this is again significant against heparin, citrate, and ACD. Again, exactly reversed to what Professor Hanss had told us. Finally, we used the single cell rigidometer (Fig. 1.24). Here we measure with about 7 mm water

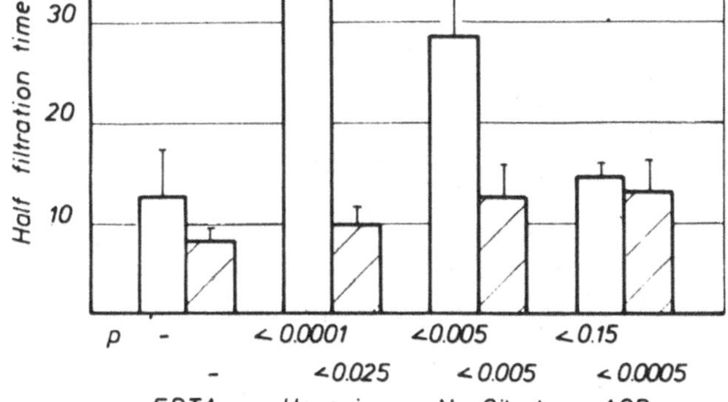

Fig. 1.22

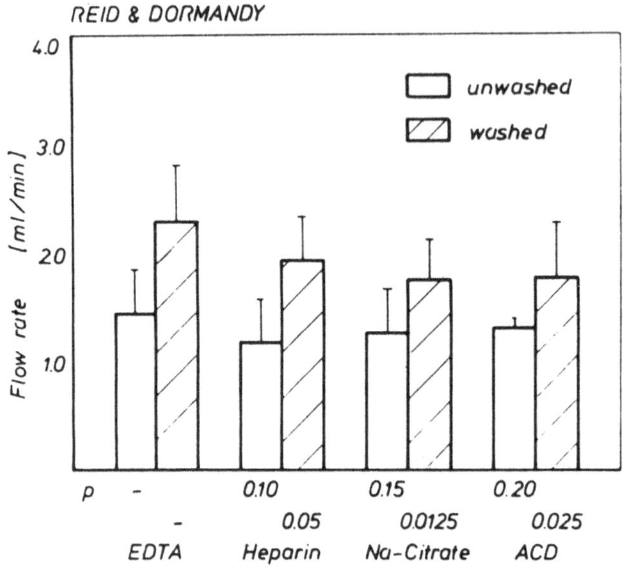

Fig. 1.23

Effect of anticoagulants on mean passage times of human RBC
(t_m, $\bar{X} \pm S.D.$, n = 33), pore ∅5,0 μm, l = 25 μm, ΔP = 70 l.
Blood suspended in buffered isotonic saline (1% albumin) at Hct 0.02, anticoagulants added to buffer.

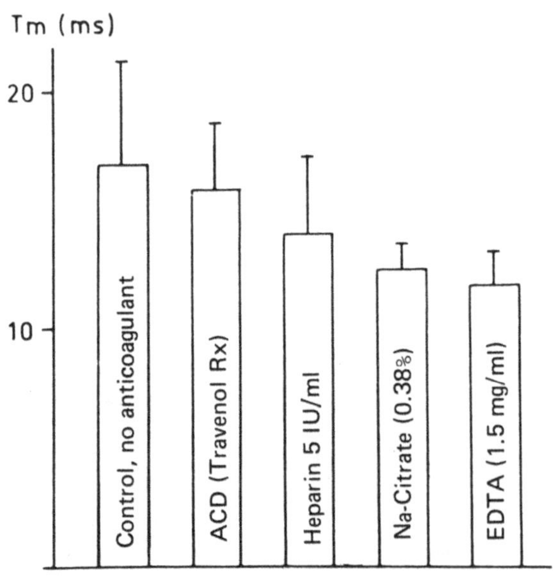

Fig. 1.24

Anticoagulant effects on RBC-pore passage time. Effect of anticoagulants in buffer.

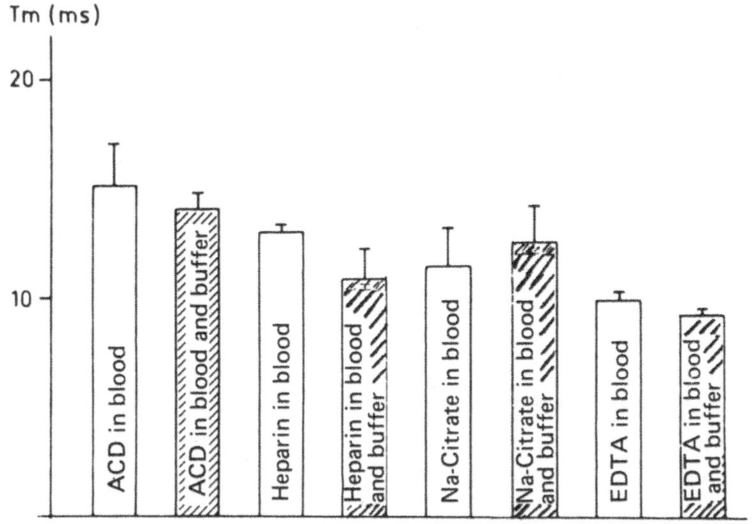

Fig. 1.25

driving pressure. The pore length is about 25 μm and the diameter 5 μm. We added blood to each anticoagulant and then put it into buffer (containing glucose and 0.25% human serum albumin). Again, EDTA has the shortest mean passage time. In a second series of experiments we not only anticoagulated the blood but also put the respective anticoagulant into the buffer and again you see (Fig. 1.25) there is essentially no big difference, the only slight increase in mean passage time seems to be exerted by sodium citrate. Although of borderline significance, statistically, we don't consider this to be biologically significant.

So we are forced to believe that in fact EDTA does something and, as I showed in Fig. 1.20, what EDTA does is to change the distribution of the cells. What we are now doing is to take half a litre of buffer and simply drop blood into that to dilute it sufficiently so there is no clotting since what we need is a control in which no anticoagulant is added at all.

P.G. Comments?

P.L. I have one question. When you said you diluted your blood samples in buffer, what was the dilution and how long was there between when you diluted the blood and when you filtered it? If we dilute cells in buffer and leave them they just won't behave the same after 15 minutes.

H.S-S. I think it is impossible to do this experiment within 15 minutes but we do it within two hours. I think we have to look at this in more detail, however. Do you have any evidence that this sort of change is counteracted by EDTA?

P.L. I don't know.

M.H. I think there may be a difference between the single cell rigidometer and the filtration apparatus because the shear stress is much lower in the former and this may be a reason for the differences between the techniques. Secondly, we have also done an experiment, on many samples, using high dilution and no anticoagulant. This gave results that were nearer the EDTA than the heparin sample. So it may be that, in our conditions, it is heparin that has some effect on the red cell and not EDTA.

H.S-S. What you are saying is perfectly acceptable. We now have a routine version of the single erythrocyte rigidometer which represents a compromise since we want the shear stress to be as low as possible but, on the other hand, we want to do a decent number of experiments per day. We used to measure at very low shear stresses (1 mm of water) but now we use 7 mm of water, so that gives us a total time for experiments of about 20 minutes including the whole washing procedure.

M.H. And how do you prepare the suspension? Do you take the buffy coat off?

H.S-S. We take the buffy coat off.

M.H. Then you mix the whole thing and take a few microlitres?

H.S-S. Exactly, and the same for each anticoagulant.

G.L. Could I just check with Professor Hanss that he is doing the same procedure as last year, that is to sample from the mid-point of the centrifuged blood sample.

M.H. Yes.

J.D. Can I ask you a simple question. If you are going to do a study *tomorrow* on 20 patients with some disease, compared with 20 controls, and you had one machine to use, what anticoagulant would you use?

H.S-S. I'll answer this question *tomorrow*! We are at a complete loss and we're still trying to digest the information we have here. Let me tell you that the majority of the studies done by our clinical colleagues are done with heparin, simply because we could not get EDTA into the routine blood withdrawal of these hospitals and because we had to rely on blood withdrawal by the nurses. At the moment, we tend to believe that heparin is closer to no anticoagulant than EDTA, but I say this with every possible precaution.

H.M. I just want to double check, Holger, the shear stress used here was about 70 pascals which is an order of magnitude or more greater than the earlier work with Kiesewetter?

H.S-S. Exactly, but this is, as I said, for practical reasons.

A.E. Some 9 years ago we studied the influence of anticoagulants on deformability of blood in our system, which is a Millipore filter system with very low pressure. The flow rate, as measured by the volume per time as well as the number of red cells passing through the filter during this time, was highest in heparin, low in citrate, and lowest in EDTA. And then we compared non-anticoagulated blood with these three anticoagulants and we found very close correlation between non-anticoagulated blood and heparin, whereas EDTA showed lower values. That means lower numbers of EDTA red cells pass the filter during a given time of 5 minutes; they are more rigid.

H.S-S. That is exactly the opposite of what we found, we find them less rigid.

P.L. A general comment. We have been talking about the ideal storage time and anticoagulant. Obviously the purpose of this was to find the optimal conditions for the study of red cell deformability. I would like to make a suggestion that could be useful in terms of standardising what each of us is measuring with different techniques. Could we not get together and define storage and anti-coagulant conditions that would provide a uniform test material? In other words, how could we all get the same poorly deformable cells? For example, we could store whole blood, in heparin or EDTA, for 24 hours at 4° C and this gives a fairly reproducible test material. This is obviously much longer than when we do a real test on a patient. If this seems like a reasonable suggestion then we could work at defining storage time and other conditions in a given anticoagulant in order to provide a test material that we could all use. I am not suggesting any particular storage conditions, I think it can be worked out between different people, but it is a suggestion I wanted to make.

G.A.M. Two points. The first is, of course, to remember the general aim. That is, not comparing temperatures or storage time or anticoagulants but studying what is happening in disease states or in physiological states or under pharmacological stresses. We must all remember that the key problem is to be comparable, whatever the storage time or anticoagulant or temperature – we must always compare patients with normals under the same conditions. In the literature, authors are very precise as to anticoagulants but they don't state how long the delay was between sampling and measuring. Usually a general order of idea is given (i.e. around two hours), but I think it is important to insist that, even for time delay, means and standard deviations are calculated.

The second point concerns heparin versus EDTA. I didn't hear many comments made on the fact that EDTA is a calcium chelating agent, whereas heparin is not. Isn't that a crucial point when we have known for years that calcium is such an essential part of red cell deformability?

A.E. When using heparin, one has to stress two important points. The first is that heparin loses its anticoagulant activity with time. If you anticoagulate for a long time then you need a very high concentration of heparin at the beginning. It is known that heparin, at least in whole blood, but not in a washed erythrocyte suspension in buffer, has an aggregating effect which may influence results in filtration techniques using a low pressure gradient or low shear rate. If we are able to measure the filtration of red cells within one hour then there is no problem, but if we have to measure after 6 hours, or even longer, then heparin is not a very good anticoagulant.

M.H. We have often studied overnight refrigerated blood samples and sometimes they are very very stiff by the next day but sometimes they are moderately stiff, so it is not a reproducible way of having stiff cells. I propose that a simpler, and more reproducible, way could be to reduce or increase the osmotic pressure of the buffer.

The second comment is on calcium. We routinely use calcium in our buffer because we thought it would be better to have a physiological level of calcium, sodium, potassium and glucose. We have made experiments with EDTA samples, with or without calcium in the buffer, and could not show any difference.

S.F. When we study differences between heparin and EDTA, using whole-blood filtration, then we see with the microscope a lot of microaggregates of red cells or platelets with heparin and with EDTA. Then if we increase the amount of anticoagulant, we have the impression that the difference between the anticoagulants is minimised. Also, when we use a double quantity of EDTA, we have better reproducibility of the method. This is a simple suggestion from our experience.

H.S-S. Could I add just one final technical comment? At the moment, new forms of heparin are being produced and if we decide that heparin should be used we would have to look into the details of the production process and at the different types of heparin in the various countries.

P.G. I think we should now have John Stuart's summarising statement.

J.S. So many of the things we have discussed this morning are interrelated that we could easily go round and round in circles. We clearly need to deal with one point at a time.

I think we have established that when we wash and then suspend red cells in a buffer, we should test these cells within minutes of making that suspension. Pierre Leblond's point that you have got to be very careful what you resuspend the cells in is also important. Brecher *et al.*, in 1961 (Annals of the New York Academy of Sciences, *99*, 242–261) showed that, even when you resuspend red cells in normal saline, you can get changes in cell size. I think that if you study red cells in suspension, then you should put your cells through a Coulter Channelyzer to make sure that the buffer does not produce a subpopulation of large cells.

The ideal is, of course, that there should be no delay from venepuncture and that there should be no anticoagulant. But we must accept a time delay unless we do all our experiments in the wards. Since the effect of time delay depends on the storage temperature and the anticoagulant, we can't answer the question on time delay until we have answered the questions on anticoagulant and temperature. So we have to consider these first. We have asked ourselves this morning which one of the three anticoagulants (EDTA, heparin or citrate) we should choose. The answer seems to depend on which filtration system we use in the laboratory. If it is a whole blood system, with contaminating platelets and white cells, then we should use EDTA. If it is a washed red cell system, with some remaining white cells, then I think you also have to use EDTA. No one has published any data on the effects of these three anticoagulants on the filtration of red cells alone and I think that is the crucial experiment which has to be done. I am sure that Professor Chien will say 'that's fine, but you should also do the same experiment on a white cell suspension to see the effects of anticoagulants on white cells'.

At the moment we probably have to use EDTA with its disadvantage that it will chelate the calcium on the outside of the red cell membrane. It does not seem to go into red cells because of its strong electronegative charge. Once a leucocyte-free system has been developed then we can go on to study heparin. The problem with heparin is, which heparin or fraction to use? There are also problems with heparin batch variation. So that all has to be standardised.

The final problem is temperature. We have talked a lot about the Na^+/K^+-ATPase. The important thing to know about cation pumps, it would seem, is the speed with which they are inhibited at 4° C and the speed with which they warm up again to the working temperature. We should also look at the effects of temperature on red cells, on white cells, on platelets, and also on the plasma. At present, the suggestion is that we should avoid storage at 4° C until one is sure that any intracellular cation changes are reversed in the warm-up time before filtering starts. Finally, it would seem important to standardise the temperature at which filtration is performed each day, ideally with a water jacket of some sort. If not, the working temperature should be recorded because a 5° C swing may be sufficient to affect the filtration rate by up to 10%.

SESSION 2

Shear stresses and haemolysis in filtration tests

P.L. To make a very short introduction I would like to remind you all of a few points that were mentioned in the summary of last year's meeting. You may remember, with respect to shear stresses, that there was and still remains a significant problem in comparing our various techniques because they work at different shear stresses. It was agreed, you will recall, that the least that we could do in the future was to state clearly what the shear forces were in the systems that each of us were using, because we all know what differences this can make. Another point had to do with the situation *in vivo*, where actual shear stresses probably never exceed something in the vicinity of 15 Pascals, yet we all know that *in vitro* filtration systems in general work at much higher shear forces. It was agreed that efforts should also be made to decrease the shear forces employed in filtration devices below the level of 100 Pascals, for fear that above such numbers one might enter into a different problem caused by red cell fragmentation and haemolysis.

During this session we shall first discuss the question of how filtration systems can be modified to function at shear stresses of 100 Pascals or less and Dr Lowe is first going to make his comments on this. Next we will hear Professor Skalak's presentation entitled 'Two-dimensional model of red cell flow into small pores'. Lastly, we will hear from Dr Herbert Meiselman about how to cause haemolysis in filters and hopefully learn how to avoid this consequence after hearing what he has to say.

P.G. Dr Lowe then.

G.L. This first slide (Fig. 2.1) just recaps upon what Pierre was saying. It is from the unpublished paper of Schmid-Schonbein and Meiselman, summarised in the report of last year's meeting, which indicates that the physiological calculated shear stresses *in vivo* reach no more than about 15 Pascals and that it is possible to calculate the expected shear stress for Nucleopore filter systems. If you know the pore geometry, you can work out the shear stresses in various systems and these of course vary from very small pressures to very high pressure with calculated shear stresses going from somewhere within the physiological range to values which greatly exceed it. As Pierre just said there are two main problems to having a high-shear system: one is of course haemolysis which has been shown to occur when you get to a certain range of shear stresses, but also equally important is the fact that with high-shear systems, one may miss subtle changes in red cell deformability. Herb Meiselman for instance has shown that if you use drugs that induce changes in red cell shape (e.g. chlorpromazine) you can observe a decreased erythrocyte deformability at physiological shear stresses, but if you expose the treated cells to higher shear stresses, they appear to act normally. For these reasons, it appears desirable then to try and reduce the shear stresses, and I will briefly show you what we have been doing recently in Glasgow. We use a system similar to that described by Pierre and others, which is a washed-cell positive-pressure flow system. We first filter the buffer and next, through the same membrane, we filter the cell suspension at low haematocrit, and record the pressure drop across the filter. The lower part of this slide (Fig. 2.2) summarizes the kind of pressures and calculated shear stresses that were shown in Pierre's paper. If you filter the buffer alone you get a mean pressure of about 3.8 mm of mercury; after adding the cell suspension, you observe an initial rise to about 4 mm Hg, due to the cells starting to go through the relatively unblocked filter and, with time, there is a progressive increase up to a final pressure of about 8 mm Hg after 10 minutes. Calculated maximum shear stresses in such a case vary from about 40 to 70 Pascals, which is perhaps more physiological than in many other previously described systems, but still somewhat above the physiological range. Bearing in mind the considerable scatter, particularly with pathological red cells, haemolysis might well occur. What we have done is to try and decrease the calculated shear stresses in a similar system, first by reducing the flow rate (from 3 ml/min to 1.5 ml/min) and by also reducing the flow time down to 6 minutes in order to minimize the time-dependent increase in pressure. We have finally increased the pore diameter to 5 microns

---

Maximum wall shear stress

1) In vivo Highest in terminal arterioles and capillaries

τ_w = 5–15 Pa (50–150 dyn/cm^2)

2) In Nuclepore filter systems

$$\tau_w = \Delta P \times \frac{\text{pore radius}}{2 \times \text{pore length}}$$

= $\Delta P \times 0.07$ for 3 μm pore filters
$\Delta P \times 0.11$ for 5 μm pore filters

In various systems,

ΔP 5 mm H_2O → 200 mm Hg

τ_w = 10 → 3,000 Pa

(100 → 30,000 dyn/cm^2)

Fig. 2.1

instead of 3 microns using a single batch of Nucleopore filters. The next slide (Fig. 2.3) shows the sort of pressure readings which we are getting in comparison to the original system. The pressure generated by buffer alone is now down to about 1 mm of mercury and we use only filters which fall within the 90% range. In a population of 54 normal subjects, the initial pressure of the cell suspension when back-extrapolated to the time when cells are just starting to go through the filter, is 1.15 mm Hg, for a calculated shear stress of 17 Pascals, just above the physiological maximum of 15. The ratio of the initial pressure to buffer pressure is very comparable to that of the previous system and with a similar range. There is about a two-fold range in normal subjects which we cannot relate to age, sex or smoking habit and we would agree with Pierre's suggestion that this probably reflects the imprecision of the method rather than true variation between subjects. After 6 minutes we obtain a final pressure of about 3 mm of mercury when the shear stress is now up to about 40 Pascals, again with at least a two-fold, if not three-fold range now. So it would seem that with cells from normal subjects we are now always staying below 100 Pascals, and to test for haemolysis we have simply measured haemoglobin in the supernatant before and after filtration. In the 20 samples tested so far, we have been unable to detect any haemoglobin, and this would be consistent with the predicted low shear stresses.

In conclusion it does seem possible to reduce the calculated shear stress towards the physiological range and thus to minimize overt haemolysis. One problem is related to the sensitivity of the pressure instrumentation which we are

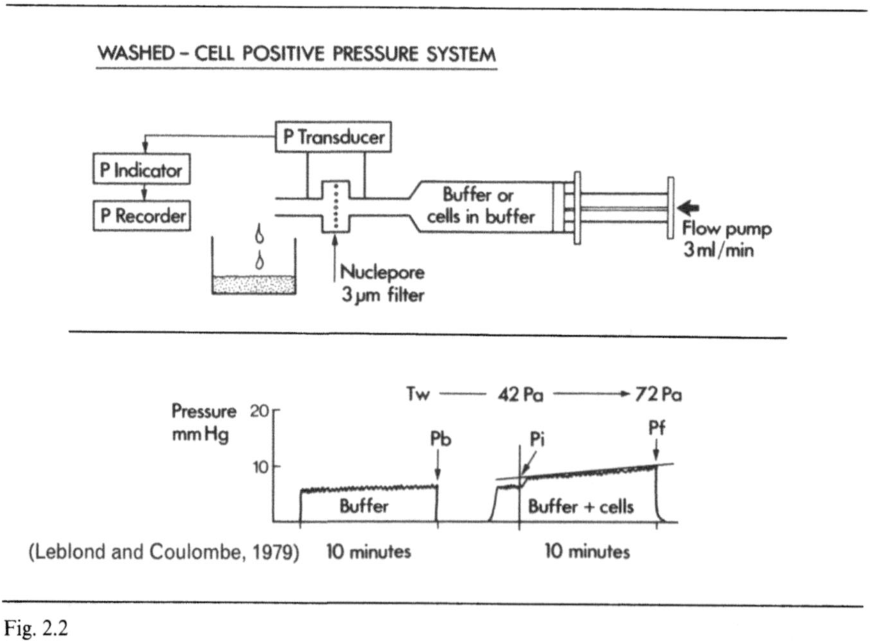

Fig. 2.2

	Leblond and Coulombe, 1979	Lowe and Anderson, 1982
P buffer	3.8 mm Hg (85% 2.5–5)	1.0 mm Hg (90% 0.6–1.4)
Normal subjects	n = 88	n = 54
Mean Pi	4.45 mm Hg	1.15 mm Hg
Initial τ_w	42 Pa	17 Pa
Pi/Pb	1.17 (1.0–1.8)	1.15 (1.0–2.0)
Mean Pf	7.75 mm Hg	2.87 mm Hg
Final τ_w	72 Pa	43 Pa
Pf/Pb	2.04 (1.4–2.9)	2.87 (1.3–3.9)

Fig. 2.3

dealing with and this may account for some lack of precision in the method. People were being rater coy about their coefficient of variation this morning. I will be quite honest and say that, on repeated studies of subjects performed on the same day we have observed up to a 30% variation in what we think we are primarily interested in, i.e. the ratio of P_i to P_b, or initial relative resistance of cells going through the membrane. And of course it is also possible that with pathological samples, haemolytic anaemias for example, because of increased blockage we might obtain higher pressures, and obviously higher shear stresses.

P.G. Thank you very much.

P.L. Gordon and I, as you know, use very similar techniques with one important difference: I use 3 micron-diameter pores instead of 5 micron. As you can see on this slide (Fig. 2.4), we also have decreased the calculated shear stress in our method to a range of 20 to 40 Pascals, mainly by decreasing the flow rate and by using phosphate-buffered saline (with added glucose) instead of Tris buffer as we did before. As expected, we saw no free haemoglobin nor LDH release in the filtrate. We also looked at echinocyte formation as a possible indicator of mechanical membrane damage, and did not see any in this case, whereas we observe up to 30% echinocytes in cells filtered at higher shear stress through similar membranes.

J.S. As that slide goes off, could you just repeat your statement about the PBS plus glucose giving a lower reading than Tris?

P.L. Yes. With normal red cells, if we use phosphate-buffered saline with 5% glucose added as a washing and suspending medium, we observe a lower resistance to filtration than with the 10 mmol Tris-NaCl buffer. As I will show you later, this difference is even more apparent if we use the smaller, 13 mm diameter membranes than the 25 mm diameter ones that we have always used.

G.A.M. A first question to the physicists. We are all very influenced by Sutera's paper saying that the shear stress in capillaries is very low, between 30 and 80 dynes per cm^2. Are we absolutely sure that, in certain patients, in certain

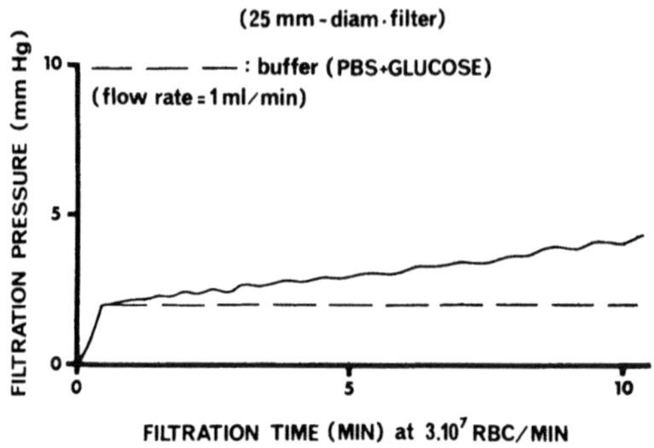

Fig. 2.4

conditions, there cannot be a turbulent flow, in capillaries even with such a low Reynold's number? When we look at P.I. Brånemark's films, for instance, when he induces occlusion and then removes the occlusion, we can see waves in all sorts of directions in the capillaries. Isn't there something eventually happening in capillaries where there could be a transiently high shear rate? My second question is more of a comment. I feel that haemolysis is not a problem in our method, working with 10% haematocrit in Tris buffer, whether we use heparin or EDTA as the anticoagulant. We are getting very high shear stresses, from 2200 to 3600 dynes/cm^2 and we have seen no haemoglobin nor LDH release. So even at shear stresses above 3000 dynes/cm^2 I think that the problem of haemolysis is perhaps not existing.

S.C. I would just like to show a couple of slides that you probably have seen before. The first (Fig. 2.5) shows that the shear stress can be simply calculated from the pressure drop, and that with a 20 cm of water pressure drop, the shear stress across a 5 micron pore-diameter filter can be quite substantial. The second point I would like to make is in relation to the problem of haemolysis. This slide (Fig. 2.6) is taken from our earlier paper on the effect of pressure change on the release of haemoglobin. This is the fraction of intracellular haemoglobin released into the medium as we filter red cells suspended in buffer through different size pores. With the 2.2 micron pores, you see that there is a large amount of haemoglobin being released when the pressure is elevated above a few mm of mercury. But as you increase the pore diameter, for example as you reach the 5 micron pores, then even with very high pressures corresponding to shear stresses much higher than 10,000 dynes/cm^2, only a very small fraction of the haemoglobin is released. This means that, at the shear stress that are commonly utilized, there should be virtually no haemoglobin released. It has been pointed out that potassium release may be a more sensitive index of haemolysis. We have studied potassium release, and as you can see on the next slide (Fig. 2.7), we can

Estimation of wall shear stress (τ_w) in filtration

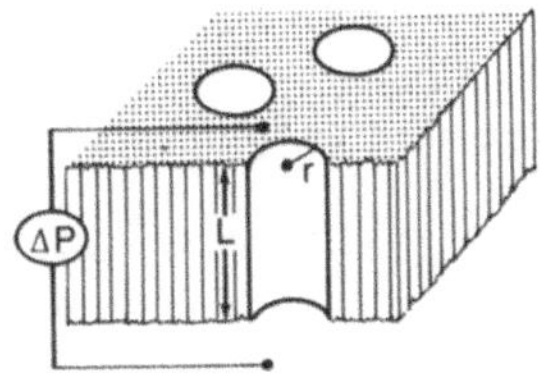

$$\tau_w = (\Delta P)\frac{r}{2L}$$

For polycarbonate sieves with 5 μm pores.

$$\frac{r}{2L} = \frac{2.5\ \mu m}{2 \times 12.5\ \mu m} = 0.1$$

ΔP $= h\rho g = (h\ cm\ H_2O) \times 1\ gm/cm^3) \times (981\ cm/sec^2)$

$\simeq 1000h\ dynes/cm^2$ (h in cm H_2O)

$\therefore \tau_w$ $= (\Delta P)\frac{r}{2L} \simeq 1000h \times 0.1 = 100h\ dynes/cm^2$

For $\Delta P = 20\ cm\ H_2O, \quad \tau_w \simeq 2000\ dynes/cm^2$

$\Delta P = 1\ cm\ H_2O, \quad \tau_w \simeq 100\ dynes/cm^2$

Fig. 2.5

release almost all of the intracellular potassium if we use a small filter and high pressure. The point is however that the shape of the curve is not that different, so if you can detect haemolysis with potassium, you can also detect it as well with haemoglobin. The next slide (Fig. 2.8) shows the very striking dependence of this phenomenon on the pore diameter. If you choose any particular index of release of potassium or haemoglobin, then look at the pressure required to produce this index (in this case, 20% of intracellular haemoglobin), and finally plot the

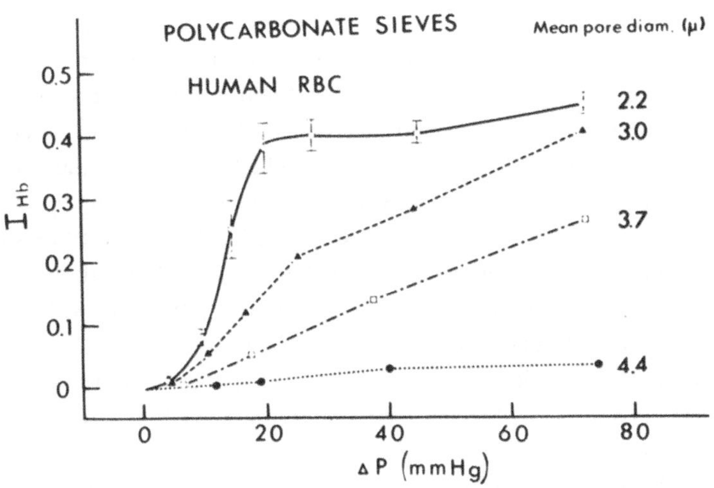

Fig. 2.6

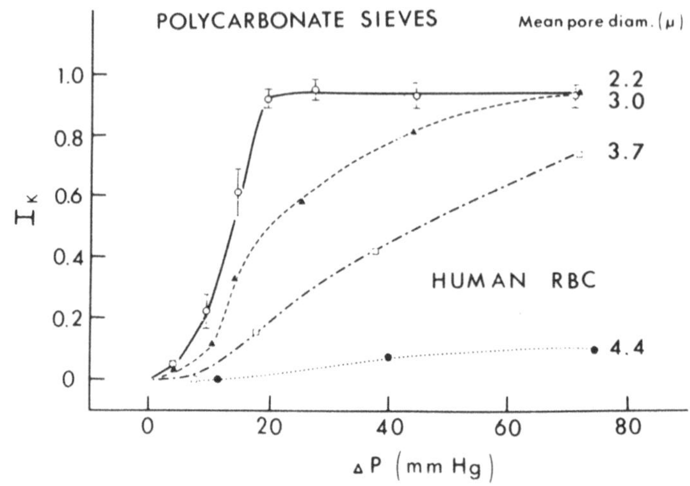

Fig. 2.7

pressure against the pore diameter, you will see that with small pores you need very little pressure, while if you increase the pore diameter you need higher and higher pressure. For 5 micron-diameter pores for instance you need much higher pressure to produce haemolysis than with the 3 micron, and this is probably one of the reasons why people are switching over to the 5 micron from the 3 micron membranes to avoid the problem of haemolysis occurring with the smaller pores.

R.S. I wanted to answer Dr Marcel's question about turbulence in the capillaries. I think a true turbulence in the capillaries is not possible because the Reynold's number is so low that instability due to inertial effects cannot really occur. But what you can have and do have is a highly unsteady viscous flow, meaning that the shear stress in capillaries is changing in time and probably in space. In one of Brånemark's movies, you see a red cell squeezing by a white cell attached to the wall of the capillary, and that red cell seems to be experiencing some very high shear stresses. In the filters that we are talking about here I also think that the red cell sees a very unsteady flow: it approaches with a very low velocity, it speeds up very rapidly to go through, it probably has to bend over the edge and then, at the exit, it does the reverse. At the microscale, therefore, flow is very unsteady and in fact the peak shear stress could be 2, 5 or even 10 times the average shear stress that we are computing.

H.S-S. With respect to haemolysis, we have some new data, presented last year in Tokyo, showing, in a very fast rotational resistometer that even if one has very high shear stresses but short exposure times, the red cells are ideally suited to

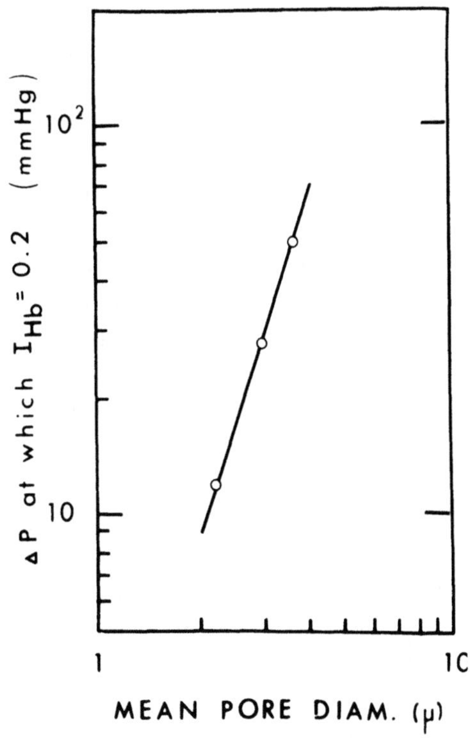

Fig. 2.8

cope with these. From what Prof. Skalak just said, in the filtration tests we are talking about here, the cells are just not exposed long enough to high shear stresses to really give and I think it is for this reason that we can most likely explain why one does not find haemolysis.

P.T. I would like to briefly mention the efforts which we have made to reduce the shear stress in our filtrometer system. In our instrument there is a non-stationary shear stress which diminishes exponentially towards zero, and it is now possible to start at considerably lower levels by decreasing the volume of suspension submitted to filtration. We can also decrease the shear stress by superimposing several discs of filter paper within the filter holder so as to reduce considerably the length of the capillary path or microscopical tube through which red cells have to pass. I will present some data on this tomorrow during Session 5.

P.G. Shall we then move on to the next presentation by Professor Skalak?

R.S. Last year I gave some elements and formulas of a macroscopic theory of filter flow and Dr Chien discussed some experimental data. This year, as I understand you already received the three papers to be published soon in *Biorheology*, my talk and Dr Chien's talk will again be correlated to bring the theory and the experiments up to date along these lines.

The first slide (Fig. 2.9) is really an overview of our theory and here, we simply have defined some vocabulary to talk about it. To begin with, we take resistance 'R_0' with plasma only, using the plasma viscosity and Poiseulle's law. The value is what leads of course to the resistance measured with the suspending fluid only, and the rate of discharge through one pore under a pressure 'P' is equal to P divided by this R_0. Now if there is a red cell in the pore at a given time, the velocity is lower and we take that into account by introducing a factor called β_1. β_1 is greater than 1 so that the resistance β_1 R_0 of course is greater and the velocity is lower when a cell is present in the pore. For white cells we just gave it a subscript 2. Now it becomes necessary to keep track of what is happening in all the pores because this results in some very interesting effects which I think most

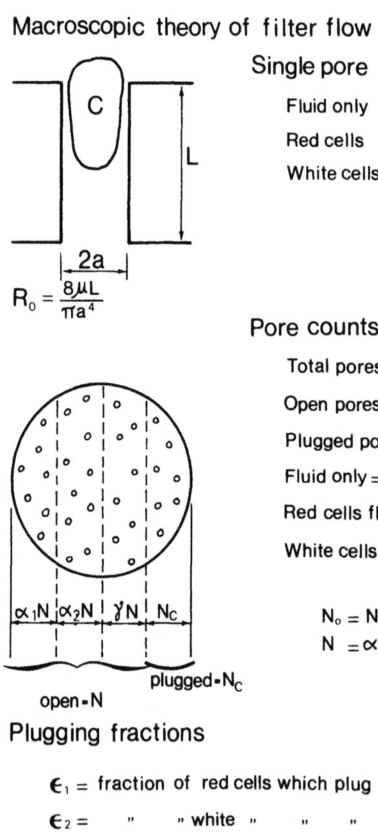

Fig. 2.9

of you can already appreciate. If you have a total number of pores N_0 at a given time, only some lower number than N_0 will represent the open pores, since there will also be some plugged ones that we call here N_c. The plugged ones are those into which there is a white cell sitting, or a clump of red cells, or a platelet aggregate, or whatever. Now, of the ones that are open you then have again three possibilities. You may have fluid only, you may have a red cell passing through the pore or you might also have a white cell. In this theory, which is for dilute suspensions, we only allow for one cell into one pore at a time. Alpha represents the fraction of pores occupied by a flowing cell as it also occurs in Dr Hanss' formula. Even though the haematocrit is usually low, I think that alpha is fairly high, ranging from 30 to 90% of all available pores, and this is a strong point coming out of this theory. So much for the basic vocabulary, now let me say just a few words about some of the basic concepts and equations. You really have two equations: one is a well-known pressure-flow equation, and the second is an equation that takes into account the conservation of mass. What it means is that in such filtration systems whatever goes in must come out, or else it is stuck in the filter and we allow for that with a transient conservation of mass equation. This morning, I will talk about our efforts to define the factor 'beta 1', that is the increased resistance which occurs when a cell is present in a pore. In thinking about this I can first argue that an axisymmetric presentation of the cell into the pore is probably a very rare event because the cells arive from all possible angles and most of them probably slide in as shown on the next slide (top) (Fig. 2.10) with a tank-treading motion of their membrane, as has been shown by Holger and by Peter Gaehtgens to occur in capillaries. With Tim Secomb, when he was at Columbia, we attempted an analysis of two-dimensional tank-treading motion in a small pore. If you focus now on the middle of that slide, that is as close as we have reached to an exact analysis for this situation. In this sketch I try to give a little more definition to the concept of the 'beta', and this bears on the discussion we just had about the transient. When a cell comes into a pore, then passes through it, if you examine, say, the discharge at the mid-plane, it will mostly drop during the entrance then, as the cell moves through, it rises and when it leaves, it goes back up to plasma or buffer only. So this is a very transient phenomenon and what we are defining here is the average flow (Q_1) while the cell passes. This will give the correct mean discharge and since you have a large number of pores and since also this is a very short time, we have a very sound concept. The model which I wanted to mention to you which will be published in *Microvascular Research* soon, is this one down at the bottom. Here I turned the pore sideways because that is how we usually think about capillary flow and this is in fact a tank-treading red cell which is asymmetric. The model is two-dimensional, meaning that these are planes, and this is like a belt going around, and it is the nearest situation to the true pores in the filter that we have been able to analyse. I think for our purposes here that I should just state the model and show the

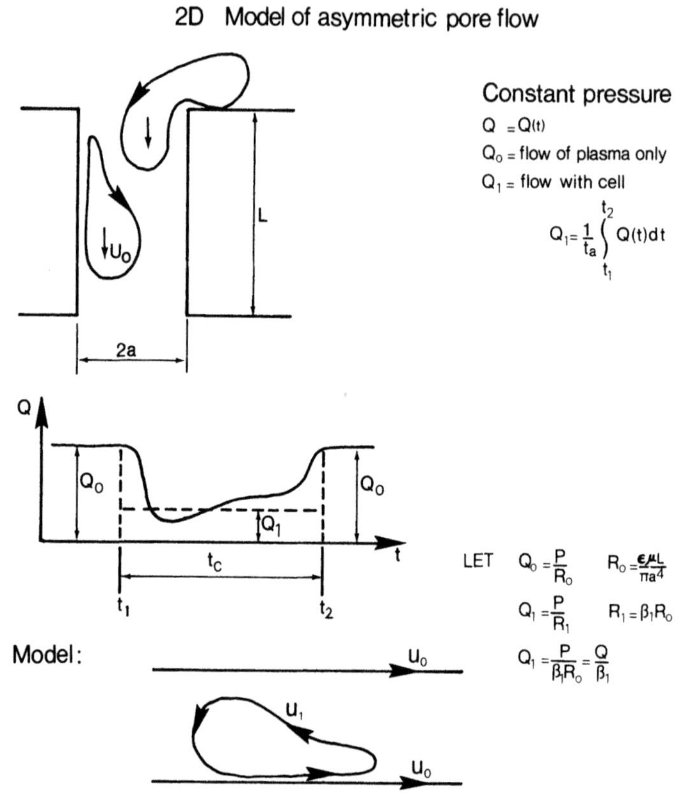

Fig. 2.10

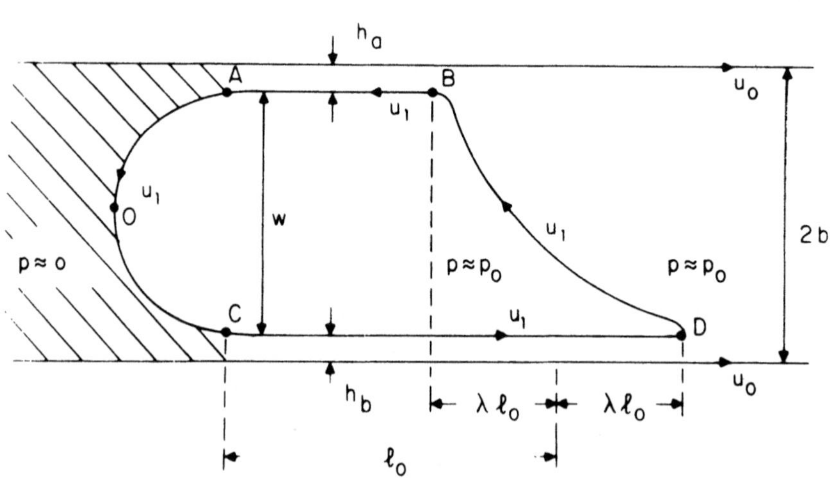

Fig. 2.11

results. The first result (next slide) (Fig. 2.11) is interesting in that the shape that you calculate for the membrane looks like a quarter circle and a straight line, but it is not exactly. Secondly the pressure in the front end of the cell rises only gradually to the rear. If we take a head pressure of 0, then the back pressure is positive and the point is that it rises just in this curved zone while, in the straight part, it is essentially constant. That gives a physical picture of how these kinds of cells work. Now, the pressure results (next slide) (Fig. 2.12). There are many things on this graph but I will refer only to this one uppermost curve which represents the pressure in a dimensionless form. And this is that parameter lambda; the symmetric cell is at 0 and it is very striking that the pressure drop appears to be lower for the asymmetric cells. Although this theory is approximate, one other thing that comes out of it is that, for a typical mid-range, the equivalent 'beta' is of the order of 5. And this is what we are using now in the computations I'll show this afternoon. I think, for the red blood cells, something certainly between 2 and 7 is about right since you cannot have much lower and it is very difficult to visualize how you could have a greater beta. Finally, I never said what controls lambda, i.e. the degree of asymmetry of the cell. I think that, in these pores, it depends on how the cell enters: some may be almost symmetric, and some may be highly anti-symmetrical. This brings up the following interesting notion: when you measure the resistance of single cells and you obtain a spectrum of values, it may not indicate any variation in the cells at all but it may

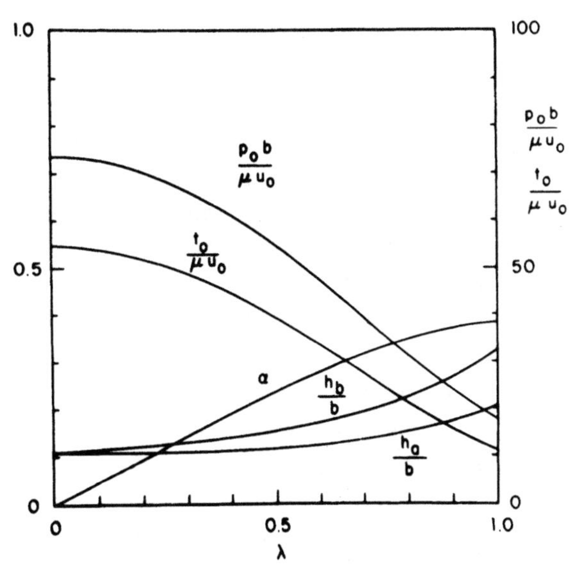

Fig. 2.12

be purely due to variation in how each cell enters the pore. For such a short pore, it is possible for perfectly uniform cells to show a distribution of resistances. This afternoon I will tell you how we incorporate the distribution in the theory. Thank you.

P.G. Holger?

H.S-S. I am not pleased with this. Let me just put up one technical point. In the SER (Single Erythrocyte Rigidometer), we have a small tube which is placed exactly above the pore, so I think, in these experiments, we have excluded the possible influence of the direction from which the cells enter the pore. However, we have a very strong feeling that the way in which the cells bump onto the wall is very decisive, and we are at the moment trying to measure two things. First, the total residence time of the cell within that pore area, in other words the approach, the passage and the exit, and this can be done optically. And then a the same time, we measure electrically the true passage time, and these two are in fact different. In other words we feel that the rolling in of the cells into the pore is a very decisive factor, and this would also explain to us why we found, two years ago, that the cytoplasmic viscosity is such a dominant feature in the phenomenon of pore passage.

R.S. For the most part I agree with the points you have mentioned. One that I would disagree with is the entry because I think that looking from above, you cannot tell how high the cell is above the wall, and unless they all come in at exactly the same height, they will suffer slightly different entry patterns. In fact, it would be extremely difficult to imagine two successive cells entering with exactly the same pattern. There are so many possibilities that to think of this in terms of a model is a difficult thing!

H.M. Just a quick question. Is it the beta-1 that increases with the more non-symmetric entry of a cell?

R.S. No, surprisingly, the beta-1 goes down, and in a way it makes sense. Suppose you wanted to slip a cell through the pore with the least amount of effort, what would you do? You would slip it over one corner and hold it against the wall. Would that not be your intuition? And if you wanted to get the worst effect you would jam it right down into the middle and try to fill up the whole pore. That is what the results are saying.

H.M. Thus, as the cell becomes more symmetric, beta-1 goes up?

R.S. That is right.

P.L. I have a piece of experimental evidence which might be interesting in relation to what you just said, and this, I may add, has been puzzling me for years. I think now that if one brings this 'entrance phenomenon' up to a macroscopic scale, it might just provide the explanation. We have compared 2 types of Nucleopore membranes, each having the same nominal pore diameter and approximately the same total number of pores; the only difference between them was the total diameter of the membrane (13 mm vs 25 mm) and, obviously, the pore density ($2.10^6/cm^2$ and $4.10^5/cm^2$). At first, we expected that the resistance to flow would be the same using either type of membrane, but what we found is what you see on the next slide (Fig. 2.13). For buffer alone, the observed resistance (at 3 ml/min) was nearly 3 times higher with the 25 mm-diameter filters (upper tracings) than with the 13 mm-diameter ones (lower tracings). However, much to our surprise, when the cells were added, we observed just the opposite situation, where the resistance is now higher in the smaller membranes than in the larger ones. Let me just add that these are original tracings obtained with the same cell suspension using either Tris-NaCl or PBS-glucose as the suspending medium. If you compare them from left to right, or vice-versa, you will see what I meant earlier when I said that we obtained a lower cell resistance by using PBS-glucose instead of Tris.

Now back to my initial problem, the only possible explanation I can think of for these differences would have to do with the geometry of the flow coming into the filter ...

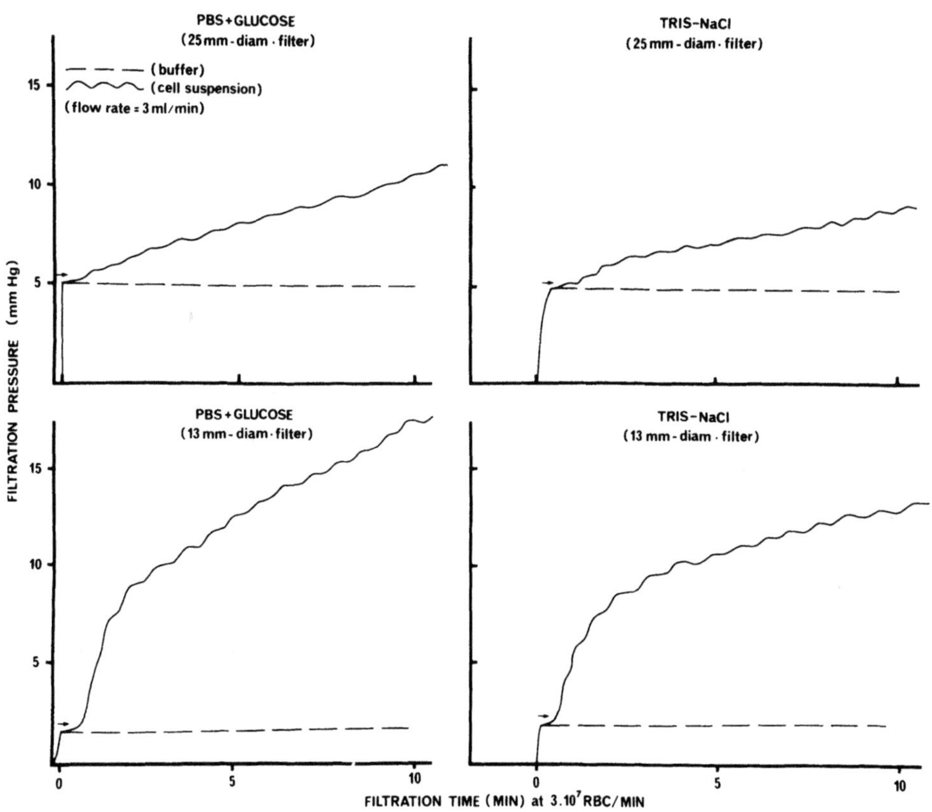

Fig. 2.13

R.S. Yes, I think it could be due to this kind of effect, namely that the flow entrance patterns for different spacings of pores will certainly be different. The extreme case is where the approach is of the same size as the pore itself, then that is a straight-through flow. If the entrance is twice as big, it will still remain mostly axisymmetric. But when you get up to 25 times as big, and have a wide area where there are no pores, then the cells will come to the wall and tend to creep along it. In that case it should also make a difference whether the filter is placed horizontally or vertically. That would be a good test to check if what you observe is an entrance effect.

P.G. Any questions or comments? If not, then I think we should move on to Dr Meiselman's presentation.

H.M. In 1971, Shu Chien and his colleagues published a paper in *Microvascular Research*, describing haemoglobin or potassium release from normal red cells and showed the relations existing between the pressure, the pore size and the degree of haemolysis observed with Nuclepore filters. Later, in 1977, Blackshear and coworkers and then, in 1980, Sutera published their theoretical analysis of the problem of haemolysis occurring through small pores. Both of them seemed to agree that you can get haemolysis if the membrane tension exceeds 10 to 30 dynes per cm when flowing through these pores. Notice that I did say the membrane tension and not the pressure drop or the shear stress. Following the suggestion of these investigators, I have therefore addressed the general question of how do deformability changes alter the haemolytic behaviour of red cells going through small pores. The experimental protocol was virtually identical to that described by Shu Chien 11 years ago: 3-micron Nuclepore filters, 25 mm in diameter, standard pore density, red cell suspensions of 1% haematocrit aspirated through the filter at various pressures, and then analysis of the material below (the supernatant) for haemoglobin, correcting for whatever haemoglobin might have been in the original suspension, this free haemoglobin was almost non-existent. The pressures that were employed ranged from 5 to 70 cm of mercury with wall shear stresses going from 400 to almost 6,000 Pascals, i.e. from 4,000 to 60,000 dynes/cm^2. So these are not a few mm of water!

This first slide (Fig. 2.14) is a familiar listing of the factors that influence red cell deformability. First, you have the extrinsic factors, including surface-to-volume ratio of the cell, and the cell shape itself, i.e. echinocytic or stomatocytic shapes, and then intrinsic factors: membrane mechanical properties (shear modulus, membrane viscosity) and the viscosity of the haemoglobin solution. We approached the question by varying as many of these factors as we could: for membrane surface-to-volume ratio we used changes in osmolality; for cell morphology we used either a stomatocytic agent (Chlorpromazine hydrochloride CZP) or echinocyte formation obtained by metabolic depletion of the cells incubated in a glucose-free Tris-calcium chloride medium at 37° C for various periods of time. To alter membrane mechanical properties, we used very low

RBC deformability

Extrinsic

- membrane surface area to cellular volume ratio (S/V)
- cellular morphology (e.g., echinocytic or stomatocytic shape)

Intrinsic

- membrane mechanical properties
- viscosity of cellular contents

Fig. 2.14

concentrations of glutaraldehyde (< 1 mmol) and for the viscosity of cellular contents, we used changes in osmolality so as to either hydrate or dehydrate the cells.

The next slide (Fig. 2.15) shows percent haemolysis in normal red cells versus the pressure driving the cell suspension through a 3-micron filter. The present study is shown by the dark circles, and the dotted line is taken from the data of Shu Chien in 1971. The insert is simply an expanded scale of the data obtained at pressure values ranging between 0 and 20 cm of mercury. It is clear that, in the low pressure region at least, there is a linear relationship between haemolysis and the shear stress, and this is in agreement with the previous data of both Shu Chien and Perry Blackshear.

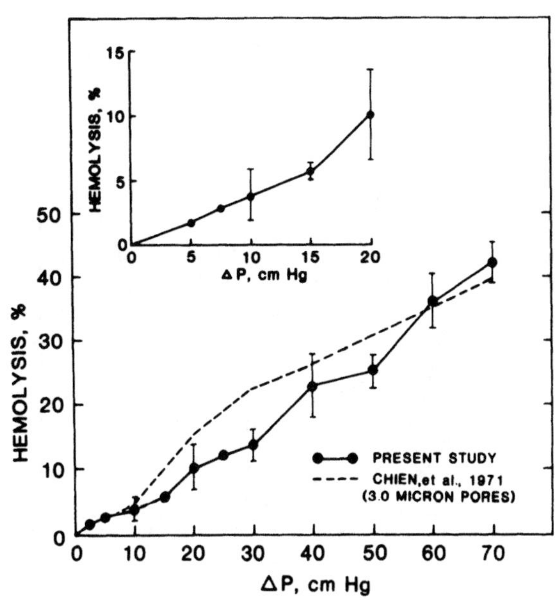

Fig. 2.15

The next slide (Fig. 2.16) shows the results obtained with cells that were either swollen or shrunken by up to about 30% using PBS of various osmolalities. Here, we have plotted percent haemolysis versus the ratio of the actual cell volume to its normal, isotonic volume. On the bottom horizontal scale, a value of 1 means isotonic and as you move left or right the cell volume is either decreased or increased by 10%, 20%, 30% or 40%. The upper scale gives the actual osmolality of the suspending medium and the four symbols are the pressures used to move the cells through the filter. From this data it is clear that if you change the cell volume, you also change its resistance to haemolysis. The minimum here occurs at isotonic conditions where the cells have a normal surface-to-volume ratio. At pressures of 10 and 20 cm of mercury, the system is very *in*sensitive to small degrees of cell shrinkage, but at higher pressures the haemolysis increases. The converse is true for swelling of the cells, that is, they are very sensitive to swelling, even for a mere 10% increase in volume. The next slide (Fig. 2.17) is just a different way of plotting the same results. Pressure drop is plotted horizontally, percent haemolysis vertically and the variable now is the volume change of the cell. At pressures of 10, 20 and 30 cm Hg, there is virtually no effect of cell dehydration. Conversely, a 5% increase in cell volume causes a significant change

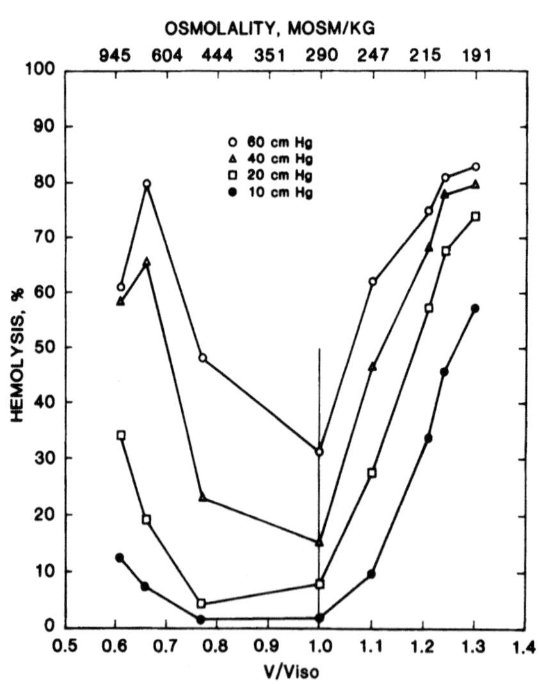

Fig. 2.16

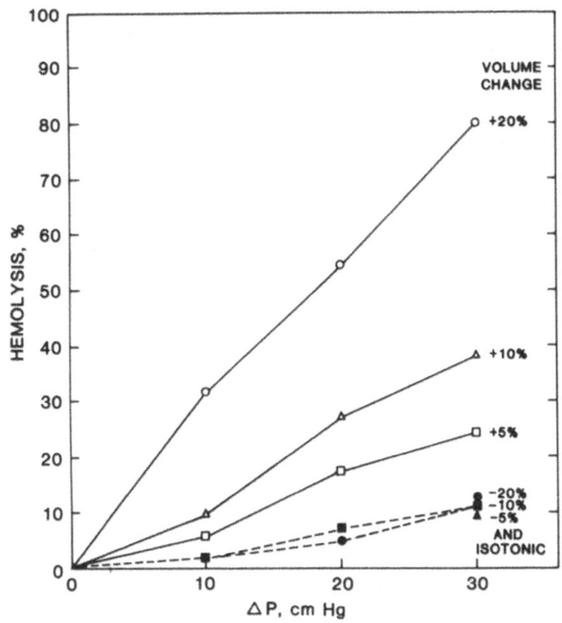

Fig. 2.17

from the isotonic condition. The system is therefore exquisitely sensitive to cell swelling but remarkably insensitive, over this pressure range, to cellular dehydration. What happens now if you change the shape of the cell by turning them into stomatocytes, using various concentrations of chlorpromazine? The next figure (Fig. 2.18) indicates that at 5×10^{-5} molar CPZ there is really no difference from the control. At 10^{-4} M, there is a large increase in haemolysis and at 5×10^{-4} M, we have 85% haemolysis at the lowest pressure examined (20 cm Hg), haemolysis remains constant thereafter, so that clearly there is an effect of CPZ leading to increased haemolysis with increased stomatocyte formation.

H.S.-S. Don't you already introduce any spontaneous haemolysis with these dramatic concentrations of CPZ?

H.M. Our measurements are all corrected for background haemolysis, but at the very high concentrations, there may have been some spontaneous haemolysis which is probably not at all physiological. Now let's examine the haemolysis behaviour if the cells are incubated in a glucose-free medium to make them become echinocytes? This figure (Fig. 2.19) shows that the difference between 0 and 4 hours of incubation is obvious, and that a plateau is reached at 24 hours.

What one sees is a progressive increase in the mechanical fragility of the cells as you incubate them longer and longer and of course there is progressive increase

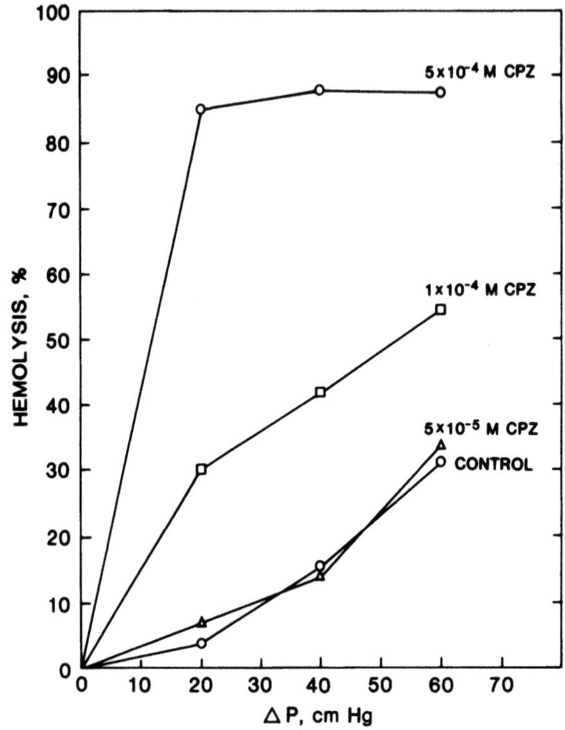

Fig. 2.18

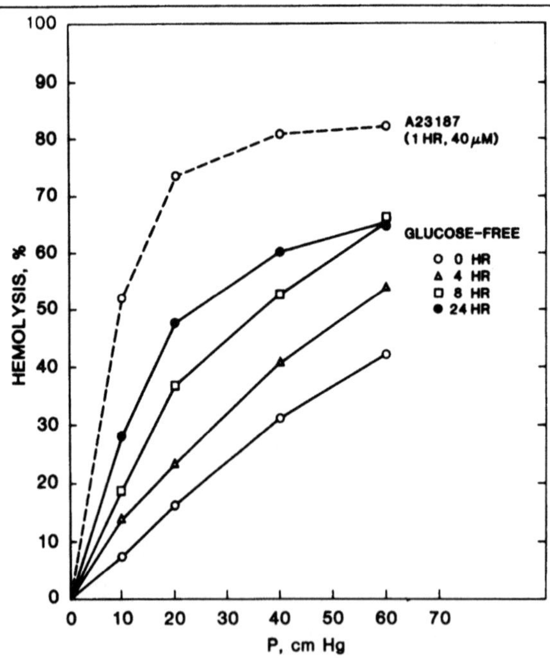

Fig. 2.19

in the echinocytic shape transformation. The relationship between ATP and time of incubation is not that dramatic; at 2 hours there is still 90% of the initial ATP; at 4 hours there is 80% left and it really takes almost 18 hours to drop the concentration of ATP to zero. So these cells at 4 hours have 80% of their initial ATP level, yet are more mechanically fragile. The dashed line at the top was obtained with cells incubated with the calcium ionofore A23187 and, as you can see, the haemolysis is higher than with any level of metabolic depletion produced by incubation in the glucose-free medium. I do not fully understand these A23187 results because the cells shrink by about 15% in the ionofore, yet I just said that there is no obvious effect with this percentage cell shrinkage in this haemolysis system. Well, what else can one do to modify cell deformability? Obviously one can treat the membrane or the cell with a cross-linking agent, such as glutaraldehyde; we used very low concentrations of 0.003% or 0.006% for half an hour. Next slide. This figure (Fig. 2.20) is not in error! In fact, the lower concentration leads to greater haemolysis in this system, and you could argue that this is because you have made the membrane more rigid but have not yet polymerized much of the haemoglobin inside, so that the situation is, in fact, like an egg shell. If you increase the concentration of glutaraldehyde slightly, you get

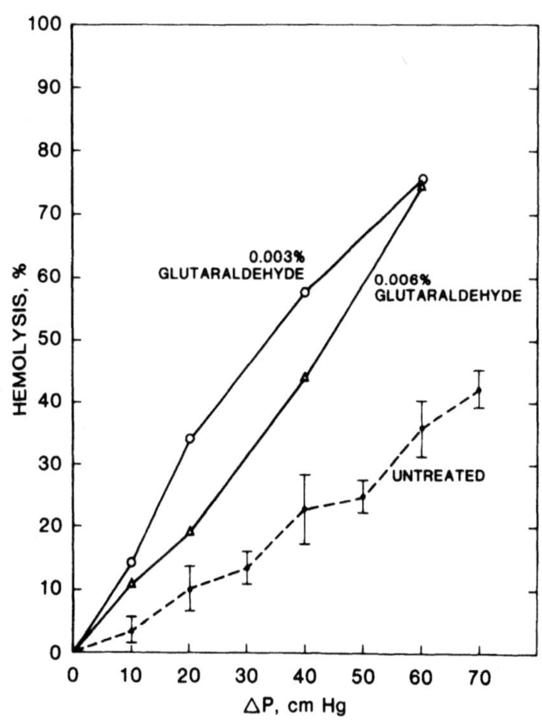

Fig. 2.20

more polymerized intracellular material, and therefore lower haemolysis.

I will now summarize all of this in three points. First of all, haemolysis can occur with normal red cells at pressures that are fairly close to those employed in some published filterability studies. At 20 cm of water for example, which is equivalent to 1.5 cm of mercury, we can calculate by linear extrapolation of our data that there could be 0.5 to 0.7% haemolysis. Secondly, for cells with a decreased deformability, which I think is what we are all looking for in these filtration studies, we have shown that they are much more sensitive to haemolysis.

The next slide (Fig. 2.21) summarizes our data on this point. As you can see, cells with a decreased deformability are all more susceptible to haemolysis than the nice fresh biconcave control cells obtained from a normal donor. And lastly, I would like to draw your attention to the possibility that even when there is no observable amount of haemolysis in the filtrate, one may be altering the flow conditions in the filter. In fact there are at least two or three reports in the literature describing what is seen on this last slide (Fig. 2.22); Dr Blackshear has described this phenomenon as a 'cluster of grapes' hanging from the bottom side of the filter and suggests that even a small amount of haemolysis can lead to this progressive accumulation of cells obstructing the pore.

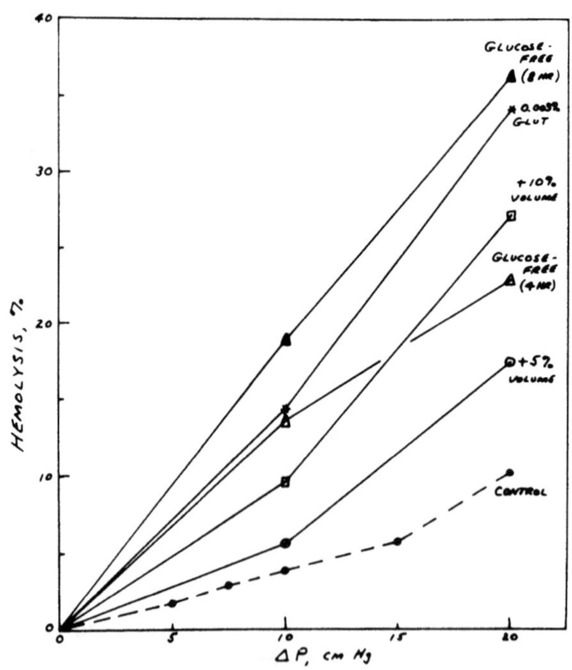

Fig. 2.21

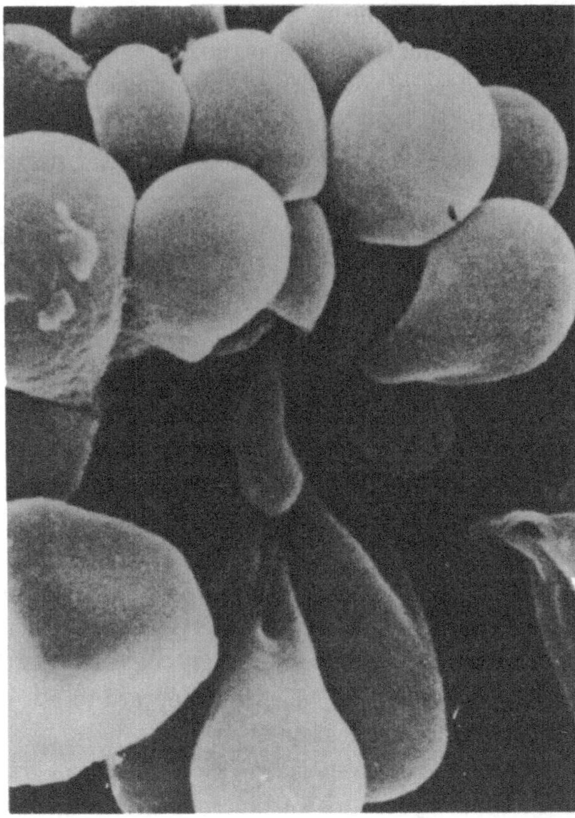

Fig. 2.22

Dr Williams in Manchester has an interesting technique in which he uses very low density Nuclepore filters where he can observe, with a microscope, cells being moved up and down the same pore.

At very small pressures of 1 to 2 mm of water, the cells appear to move without problems, but as soon as you use a slightly higher pressure, they begin to accumulate and look as if they were hanging from or adhering to the downstream edge of the pore. These observations are why I think that haemolysis can alter not only what you see in the filtrate but also the flow conditions of the filter itself. In fact I wonder if this type of adherence might occur in those kinds of filtration experiments in which the flow rate is kept constant and the pressure differential is recorded? Let's assume that maybe it does not occur with normal cells but could it with pathological cells, where the pressure rises very steeply? Perhaps such a process is happening. In summary then, I suggest that you evaluate the problem of haemolysis in your filtration systems and avoid it if possible. Thank you.

P.G. Thank you Herb. Comments, questions?

G.L. Just on your last point Herb. We have taken similar electron micrographs of filters using our more recent low pressure system and we never see that kind of bunch of grapes or whatever else you want to call them, whereas we saw them previously, when we were working at much higher shear stresses and higher haematocrits.

G.A.M. Three questions concerning the calcium ionofore. First question: were you adding any extracellular calcium? (*H.M.*: Yes). To what concentration? (*H.M.*: 2 milimolar, i.e. physiologic). Second question: were you dissolving your A23187 and all that in alcohol or DMSO? (*H.M.*: in alcohol). And third question: in your abstract, you state that 'increased intracellular calcium levels via A23187 had a profound effect'. Are you sure that it was the increased intracellular calcium? One possible way of knowing, and I am not sure it works very well, is to try and inhibit the calcium transporting effect of A23187 by nifedipine or by flunarizine to see if it is the A23187 itself which is haemolytic or if it is the calcium.

H.M. Yes (D-600), I guess, will also do the same thing, i.e. inhibit the entry of calcium and block the effects of the ionofore. As you know, calcium ionophores have fairly complex effects and I am not sure that I could do more than to merely speculate as to why this substance, which we happened to use, causes greater haemolysis than glucose-free incubation.

P.L. I just want to go back very quickly to these 'clusters of grapes'. I can tell you from experience that if you work with micropipettes, one of the worst things that can happen to you is to haemolyze a red cell in the tip of the pipette, because then the effective diameter of that pipette tip has changed, and you just have to discard it and start your experiment all over again. Another point related to the effect of such clusters in the results of filtration experiments. What you said is interesting because I have been trying to calculate, on the basis of Poiseuille's law, what the effect of a given number of white cells would be in our system, by making the simple assumption that each white cell can plug one pore. And each time, we observe a greater resistance, in our experiments, than what we can account for on the basis of the number of white cells present in the sample relative to the number of pores available on the filter. I have done the same for your system using the numbers you gave and you have the same phenomenon. So there is some degree of resistance in our system, and probably in yours too, Gordon, that cannot be explained on the basis of the simple assumption that each white cell can occlude one pore. Perhaps in the 3 micron filters one might accept the possibility that a small percentage of normal red cells cannot make it through the pores but I don't think this would be acceptable for the 5 micron filters. So, maybe these clusters, after all, are significant.

J.D. Do you have any idea what it is about the haemolysis which messes up the pores, because that is the crux of the matter, isn't it? For the amount of haemolysis you show, I mean, 1 or 2%, this would not matter in terms of losing red cells, it would only matter because it blocks the pores. What is it then about haemolysis which does that, and have you tried adding, for instance, free haemoglobin to buffer at normal pressures?

H.M. No. The only point I was making, was that if you have a tendency for haemolysis to occur you will see this 'cluster' phenomenon and you may get this progressive plugging of the filter.

J.D. What is it about haemolysis which has that effect?

H.M. Well, it is probably the same thing that Pierre has pointed out in small glass pipettes.

P.L. What you see in micropipettes is a tiny amount of what appears to be stroma or membrane that sticks to the inside wall of the tube and reduces its diameter.

J.D. My second question would be: is this not an argument against the use of constant-flow systems, where the pressure can rise, leading to a variable degree of haemolysis and therefore also a variable degree of plugging which you cannot actually measure or quantify?

H.M. What you measure with such systems is mostly plugging. I know Shu Chien has made some measurements with sickle cells for instance, where the pressures really rise dramatically and, in a general sense, what you measure is plugging, even if you don't know the exact mechanism, i.e. whether it is due to ISC_s, or to something else occluding the pores and causing other cells to stick. The most dramatic example of this, besides the micro-pipette, is in the technique developed by Williams, which I mentioned earlier. As I said, the cell moves back and forth very easily through the pore until you rise the pressure slightly; then you begin to see one-way movement only, and pretty soon there appears this 'cluster of grapes' as if something had become attached to the surface of the filter, causing other cells to stick to each other.

S.C. Herb, I think, in all fairness, that your studies take us so much farther than our earlier ones, and I am very impressed. I would just like to comment on the sticking of cells on the exit side of the filter. I think Larry Lessin probably was the first one who showed these, which he called 'bouquets' of sickle cells on the downstream side. Sickle cells, I think, are the red cells that are more prone to this kind of 'bouquet' formation, but we see this also in the case of white cells. In fact, whenever a white blood cell sticks to the filter this will encourage the formation of these grapes or bouquets on the downstream side.

P.G. Let us now open the floor for the general discussion. Let us hear your comment, Professor Hanss.

H.M. Professor Skalak told us earlier that the fraction 'alpha' of pores occupied by red cells in micropore filters should be very high, according to his theory. I don't agree with his estimate of 90%, and I think it can be much lower.

R.S. It can be low, but you would need extremely low haematocrits.

M.H. I made a rough calculation and I estimate that in the 'haemorhéomètre' for a haematocrit of 8%, alpha should be around 10%.

R.S. I will say at least.

S.C. I think the answer to that question lies in the beta value. If beta were close to 1, then the alpha should be the same as the entrance haematocrit in the feed or the reservoir. But if beta is significantly higher than 1, the higher the beta is, the greater will be this alpha. If the beta is equal to 5 the alpha can be significantly higher.

M.H. Yes, but the feed haematocrit is not very different from that in the reservoir on top, and the transit time for a volume of water equivalent to that of a red blood cell is not very much different from the transit time of the red cell itself.

R.S. Holger, are you going to agree with that?

H.S-S. I think before we have more information about the true passage-time of the cell and can substract the collision-time with the wall I would not want to stick out my neck at this time. So I think, at the moment, we have to leave this open.

M.H. But have you calculated the transit time for water volume?

H.S-S. Oh yes, and we are in the same order of magnitude as that observed for a population of normal red cells. As soon as you have abnormal cell, you must consider the existence of a retardation effect at the entrance into the pore and I would say that, in the case of many patients having poor filterability, this is what happens. There are just a small number of cells which will not enter and which form an obstacle, as if one of us here was holding that door half-shut. Only one of us does it, but all of us would have a bad time trying to get out of this room. I have very strong feelings in this direction and we are trying to do some experiments along these lines.

P.G. We all seem to be satisfied and waiting for Pierre Leblond's summary.

H.S-S. If I may ask a question to Herb before you summarize? You restricted yourself to the 3-micron filters in your experiments and, even in these, it is only in the range of pressures situated below where you have actually made your measurements that you assume there might be some shear-induced haemolysis in the conventional Reid/Dormandy or similar-type test. Have you really looked at the model that we are discussing here, in other words, do the clinicians have to fear from your experiments that there might be a significant amount of haemolysis in their tests? We have heard from Tony Marcel that there is none and I should say that we do not see very much either. But what is your own experience?

H.M. I have no experience directly below the levels of 10 or 5 cm of mercury. If I had to guess, I would say that, for normal red cells, I agree with everyone that there probably is no haemolysis at 1.5 cm of mercury or 20 cm of water. What worries me is that when we alter the cells, no matter how we do it, those haemolysis curves all rise above the control value, so that even in the low-pressure region you might have more haemolysis than what is anticipated with normal cells. But I have no data to support that.

G.A.M. Just a small additional comment on what you said. Although we are measuring haemoglobin, LDH, and whatever, the lab technicians usually have an excellent eye for haemolysis. In many cases we have not been checking the LDH after filtering a patient's blood, but nevertheless one of the first things that a technician will mention is that there seems to be some haemolysis there.

P.G. But then it is already massive, and one can see it ...

G.A.M. No, no.

H.M. I wonder how many people actually spin down their filtrate to look for haemolysis? I rather think that once you have filtered the suspension, you usually say: 'well there it is, disposable test tube, throw it out, and do the next study ...'

R.S. Besides these experiments there is also a theoretical point which I think has some bearing on the problem of haemolysis. In the resistance phenomenon, Holger is now talking about distributions and we also are looking at the theory of that. I think that the individual cells, due to their age differences if nothing else, will have a spectrum of thresholds for mechanical haemolysis so that you should not expect to find a sharp demarkation. Even at very low pressures, a certain number of cells will probably be haemolysed, perhaps one in a million, or one in 2 million and so on, but I think it will build up progressively from very low pressures if you have a test sensitive enough to detect it.

M.H. I have a few figures to give you with regards to haemolysis. We have been doing some experiments using large tubing and a pump to look at mechanical haemolysis under vibration. The vibration, I would say, increases the shear stress by about 100 Pascals, no more. Then we measured haemolysis on the cell suspension and found that we needed at least half-an-hour of vibration to obtain 0.1% haemolysis. So I think that low shear stresses for a small period of time should cause no macroscopic problem. Of course, there can always be that one cell or two, but that is another problem.

P.G. Pierre Leblond will now summarize.

P.L. I have made a short list here on my paper of what I believe we may have learned this year about these two topics of shear stress and haemolysis in filtration systems. I think it has been quite clearly expressed that, with the 3 micron-diameter Nucleopore membranes, you begin to see haemolysis at shear stresses of approximately 150 Pascals. It also stands out that with the 5 micron membranes, the risk of seeing haemolysis with normal red cells is probably much less. For abnormal cells however the risk of haemolysis happening even at those shear stresses is considerably greater, and we must therefore keep this in mind. It strikes me after having seen Herb's data, that the results he gets by measuring haemoglobin release in 3 micron membranes at very high shear stresses are, in a sense, quite similar to what we have previously observed measuring ΔP at lower shear stresses. In other words, you told us that, when you swelled the cells by simply decreasing the osmolality of the buffer, your system was very sensitive to that in terms of haemoglobin release. Conversely, when you shrunk the cells by increasing the tonicity, it was not very sensitive. Well, we observed exactly the same thing in our system, except that our end-point for measurement was ΔP and that we were working at much lower shear stresses. In other words despite the apparent differences between our two systems, we are perhaps measuring the same thing, except that we are each looking at it from a different viewpoint. This reminds me of a remark that was made in Göteborg, I think, by Professor Skalak who gave us the example of a block of concrete, and about how hard you had to smash it before it breaks, in order to examine its expected resistance under normal conditions, which may not be so severe. In any case, I think we all realize that filtration systems should be kept at the lowest possible shear stresses if one wants to stay away from the problem of haemolysis. In order to do this with the constant-flow-rate devices, one may run into some technical difficulties in measuring very small amounts of pressure, and this is something that some of us will have to continue working on. On the other hand, Paul Teitel's variable-flow-rate system is somewhat ideal in terms of shear stresses, but the problem with his approach is mainly with analysis of the results, and unfortunately not everyone can have the sophisticated computer and software that Paul has developed over the years. So, there are still some technical problems remaining to be solved and it should be interesting, in a year's time, to watch for any accomplishments in that direction. We have also heard today a number of interesting suggestions to explain the pressure differentials that we see in filters with normal as well as abnormal red cells. I think that the idea of integrating the combined effects of empty pores, of pores with white cells, or pores with red cells in transit as a function of time seems like something that will make us better understand what is really happening, because our general tendency is to visualize filtration from rather simplistic assumptions, such as each-white-cell-blocks-one-pore, and so on. Conservation of mass, as Professor Skalak put it, may too often be overlooked in our efforts to analyze our results, and a nice example of this was provided by what Herb Meiselman politely brought back to our attention as the 'cluster of grapes' phenomenon. The fact that red cells may at times adhere to each other or to the surface of the filters, and that this may have a profound effect on our measurements is certainly something that we will be more aware of in the future, although I am not sure how we can precisely analyze for this. Certainly, here lies a nice little puzzle for our mathematically-oriented friends to work on until next year!

My last comment is really intended to bring us back where we started this session, i.e. the desirability of filtering red cells at low shear stresses. I can't help but to remind you of an observation that was made a few years ago by someone working in Schmidt-Schoenbein's laboratory about the deformability of red cells that had been previously treated with Diamide in order to crosslink their spectrin. Correct me, Holger, if I am wrong, but it was said that such cells were found to be abnormally deformable only when tested at very low shear stresses, while they appeared normal at 'standard' driving pressures. Most striking to me was the fact that the same cells, when injected directly into the circulation of a healthy rat, were found to survive in a perfectly normal manner. My question is therefore: as we are attempting to make our techniques more and more sensitive to subtle changes in deformability, are we not possibly 'overshooting' to a point where we might miss some of the things that we are really interested in?

P.G. Thank you very much Pierre for an excellent summary.

SESSION 3A

Effects of haematocrit, leukocytes and platelets

P.G. We start going into Session 3A and 3B organised by Shu Chien. Session 3A will deal with the effects of haematocrit, leukocytes and platelets. We should start by calling on Dick Skalak to present his contribution.

R.S. As I mentioned this morning, in my talks today I am reviewing the theory that we started last year and that we have developed further this year. Dr Chien will give extensive experimental results, and both theory and experiments are contained in the three papers distributed earlier. The talk will go a little further in some aspects that are not in those papers.

To begin with, we define a resistance to flow of suspending fluid only through a single pore as R_0. When there is a red cell in a pore the resistance is increased $\beta_1 R_0$, where β_1 is a factor somewhere in the range 2 to 7. For white cells there is another resistance $\beta_2 R_0$ where the factor β_2 may be 100 to 1,000. To describe a plugging cell may require a very high value of beta. In the latest work, we consider both β_1 and β_2 to have statistical distributions. I think that will be the most realistic.

The equations used are pressure-flow relations and conservation of mass. In any test, every pore is subject to the same pressure drop and the total discharge is the sum of all the pore discharges. That is one equation. The other is the conservation of mass. In a steady state, the flow into the filter equals flow out of the filter. This must be true individually for the red blood cells, for the white blood cells, and for the suspending fluid. The other extreme is plugging. If there were some cells, say one of the types of the leukocytes which could not go through a typical pore at all, you would have a flow into the filter but you would not have any flow out. When that happens, the percentage of pores which are occupied by these cells goes up gradually. This shows that the α factors (the percentage of pores occupied by a given type of cell) can be functions of time depending on the relative retardation. In order to get computations going, we assume that when the pressure is first applied one forces into the filter exactly the haematocrit in the approaching flow. And the same holds for the leukocrit. But thereafter the entering white cells go more slowly and they stay longer than the red cells. For this reason the α_2 (percentage of pore occupied by the white cells) goes up. That turns out to be a very strong and dramatic effect. At very short times the red cells predominate because they are assumed to have a haematocrit of about 2–10% and the leukocrit is typically only about 0.2%. According to our results if you have 10% haematocrit in the feed reservoir, the haematocrit in the filter is about 72% after a fraction of a second. This is shown in Fig. 3.1 by the uppermost curve which is for a hematocrit of 10% and a leukocrit of 0.2% in the approaching flow. This is based on a β_1 for the red cell of 5. If you have an approaching haematocrit of the order of 27% every pore will have a cell in it or very nearly. When such high haematocrits are used, there may develop a layer of cells over the filter.

Figure 3.2 shows the percentage of the pores occupied by white cells (α_2). This rises more gradually but still takes only about a second to reach a sort of plateau. At longer times the theory will give a continued rise of pressure only if one assumes that some percentage of the white cells actually plug the pores. This is the ε, here assumed to be 0.2. That means 20% of the white cells plug. The next figure (3.3) shows the effect of plugging on the pressure p required for constant total discharge. There is a rapid initial rise which probably cannot be resolved experimentally. It is only a small fraction of a second. The later steady rise is due to plugging.

I would like now to say what we have done recently to try to make the theory more realistic. This is to have a distribution of betas. I think again for our

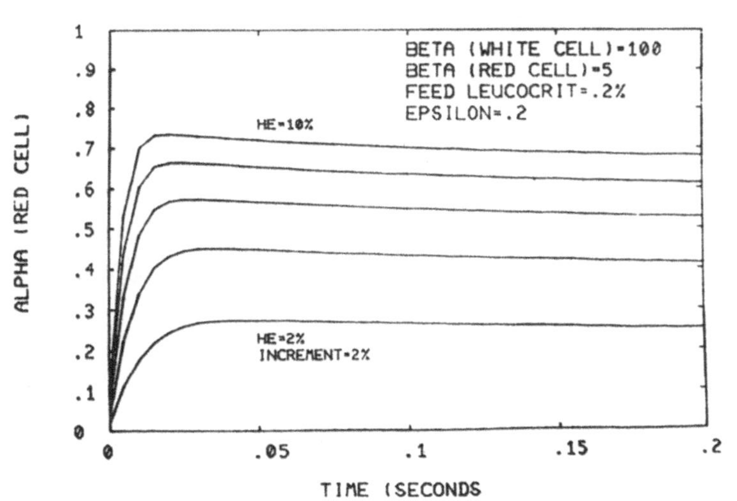

Fig. 3.1. Fraction (α_1) of pores in a 5 μm nuclepore filter occupied by red blood cells shown as a function of time. The lowest curve is for a feed hematocrit of 2% and the subsequent curves are for increments of 2% in this hematocrit. The feed leukocrit is constant at 0.2% for all cases.

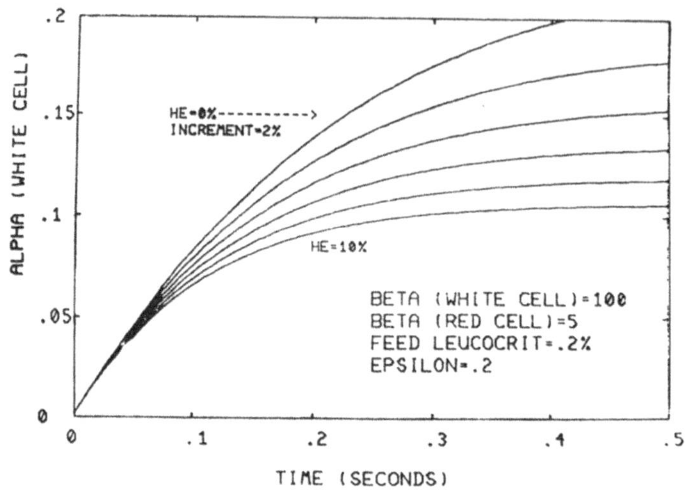

Fig. 3.2. Fraction (α_2) of the pores in a 5 μm nuclepore filter occupied by white blood cells shown as a function of time. The uppermost curve corresponds to zero hematocrit in the approaching flow (white cells only). The subsequent curves are shown for increments in the hematocrit of 2% for each curve up to 10%. These curves correspond to the same cases as in Fig. 3.1.

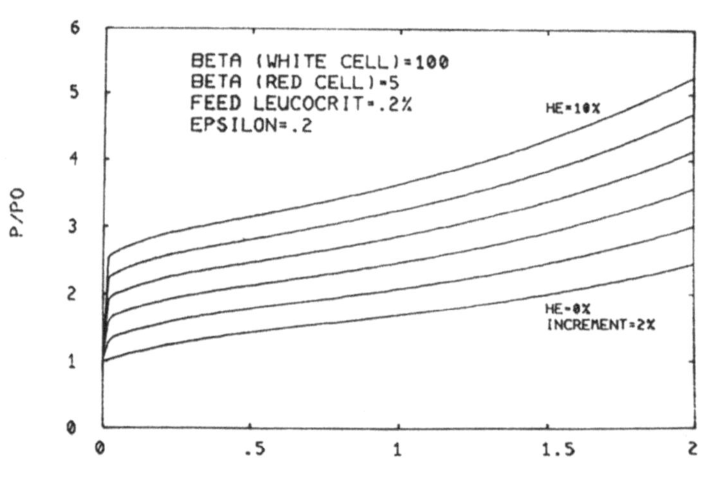

Fig. 3.3. Pressure vs. time for constant flow through a nuclepore filter of 5 μm pores for the same cases as shown in Fig. 3.2. The bottom curve is for zero hematocrit in the approach flow (white cells only). The subsequent curves are for increments in the hematocrit of 2%. The pressure P_0 is the value for the flow of the suspending fluid only with no cells present. The ratio P/P_0 indicates the influence of the blood cells.

purposes here it is sufficient just to concentrate on two variables. The first is K(β) which is a probability distribution of cells with resistance factor β in the approaching flow. This distribution should be thought of as exactly the curve as Dr Schmid-Schoenbein showed this morning. The second variable is the distribution G(β) of resistances in the filter because these are different. The slow cells have high resistance and they stay in the filter longer than the fast ones; therefore, in the filter one sees a predominance of the slow cells. In whole blood filtration it is the white cells that amplify their presence very greatly this way.

Now to be realistic we assume that K(β) is the sum of two normal distributions. The first one represents red cells and the second one represents white cells. The K(β) distribution represents the β (resistance) distribution for cells in the approaching flow. The G(β) distribution is in the filter.

The distributions for one case are shown in this figure (3.4). In the approach flow the cellular content is 98% red cells and 2% white cells. The distribution K(β) near $\beta = 100$ represents white cells but you can hardly see this K(β) distribution because it is so close to the axis. The large peak of K(β) near $\beta = 5$ represents the red cells. This kind of plot visualises the relative numbers of red and white cells in the approaching flow. In the filter the distribution G(β) shows that the red cells are somewhat reduced percentage-wise and part of the curve for white cells is more prominent. The area under the G(β) curve will be the per-

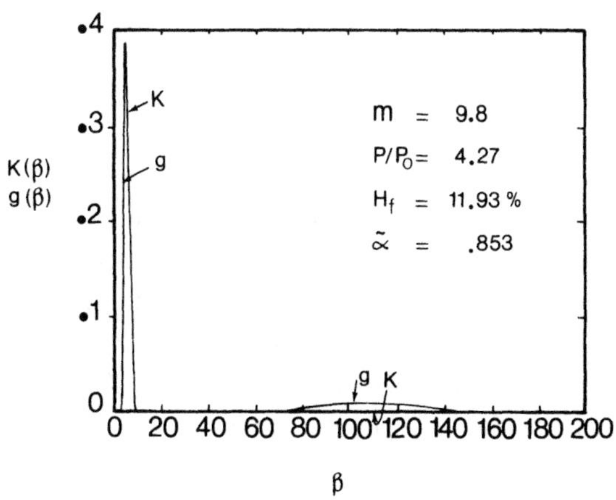

Fig. 3.4. Distributions of the resistance factor β in the approach flow (K) and in the nuclepore filter (G). The assumed distribution for K consists of two normal distributions, one for red blood cells centered at $\beta = 5$ and a second normal distribution centered at $\beta = 100$ to represent white blood cells. The distributions in the nuclepore filter are shown by the curve G which is lower than K for the red cells but much greater than K for the white cells.

centage of pores occupied by the cells. The distribution G(β) shows in a graphic way the relative influences of red and white cells.

To simulate plugging, one can specify an initial white cell distribution K(β) a small tail at high β values, meaning a very small fraction of them have a very high resistance. The slowest of them may be specified to take several minutes to go through the filter, so for any test less than several minutes they are essentially permanently plugging. This will produce a gradual pressure rise as such cells collect in the filter. The expectation is that this double type of distribution and a realistic tail on the high end of β values for white cells will reproduce the whole history of pressure that one sees in real filters. We have not yet carried out such computations exactly. At present we are able to describe such cases approximately by using a number of discrete parameters (fixed values of β for each type of cell). Dr Chien will give a number of examples and extensive experimental data. Thank you.

P.G. Should we have Shu's talk right following it and then have a joint discussion of both?

S.C. It is always a pleasure to follow Dick because he sets the stage and makes my job a lot easier. What I would like to present to you are some of the results we have obtained with Dr Emily Schmalzer on the filtration of suspension of red cells and white cells. The results have been analysed by using the approach that Dick has outlined. These studies were done on 5 μm Nuclepore filters using a constant flow technique, and the pressure was monitored with time. This slide shows four such tracings of the pressure–time curve. The two graphs on the left are the tracings obtained with 5% haematocrits but with different white cell concentrations. In the lower left tracing, when the white cell is reduced to a very low level (10/mm^3), the pressure rise initially to a level P_i indicated by the arrow, the subsequent pressure rise is not very prominent. In contrast, the upper left tracing was obtained for a suspension in which the red cell concentration is the same (5% haematocrit), but the white cell concentration is increased to 750/mm^3. There is still an initial pressure rise (marked by arrow), which can be seen much more clearly at a higher paper speed. This very short period of initial pressure rise is followed by subsequent pressure rises composed of an earlier rapid phase and a later slower phase. The two tracings on the right were obtained for suspension with relatively high white cell concentrations (500 and 650/mm^3), while the haematocrit was adjusted to either 20% (upper right tracing) or 2% (lower right tracing). Here the initial rise in pressure P_i (marked by arrow) is higher with high haematocrit and lower with low haematocrit. These effects of changing the white cell concentration and the red cell concentration on P_i will be summarised on the next two slides. After that I will discuss the effect of these cell concentrations on the slopes of the subsequent phases of pressure rise: k_1 for the earlier rapid phase and k_2 for the later slow phase.

H.M. Is there any significane to the amplitude of the pressure signal, if you

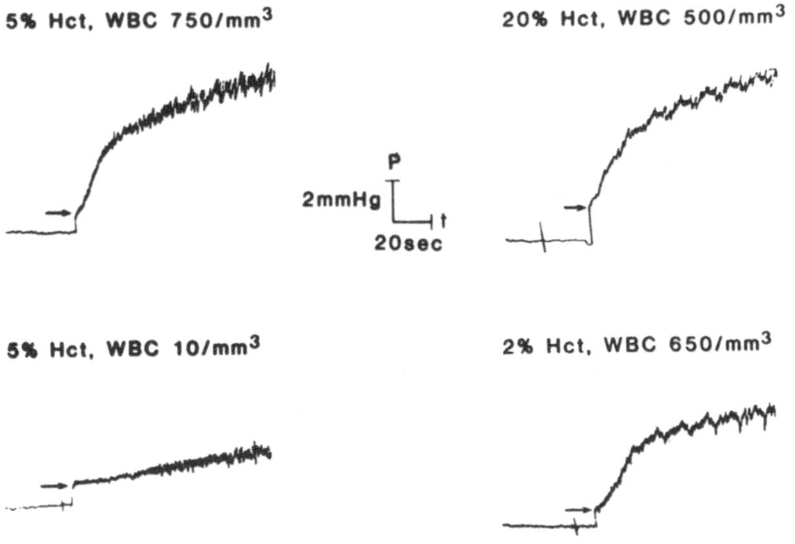

Fig. 3.5

will, noise? Is it much higher with the higher white cell count? Is there anything to that?

S.C. These are the very early recordings. The oscillations on the pressure tracing reflect the imperfection of the pump we used; therefore they are mechanical noises. Nowadays we have improved our system so that the noise is smaller.

R.S. This is mechanical noise. Not white cell noise.

S.C. Slide (Fig. 3.6). Now we will continue our discussion on the effects of white cell concentration on P_i. The initial pressure P_i is normalised by dividing it by the pressure P_0 recorded when the suspending medium, the buffered Ringer solution, was pumped through the same filter at the same flow rate. This dimensionless P_i/P_0 ratio does not show any significant correlation with white cell concentration up to 12,300/mm^3.

Slide (Fig. 3.7). The red blood cell concentration or the haematocrit, on the other hand, has a strong influence on the P_i/P_0 ratio. The data points up to a haematocrit of nearly 30% can be fitted by the regression line (drawn as a solid line). We also derive a regression equation (dashed line) which requires the curve to go through the origin of 1,0, i.e. P_i should $= P_0$ when there is no red cell. The regression equation is $P_i/P_0 = 1 + 0.074$ H where H is the haematocrit (in %). Therefore, the data indicate that P_i/P_0 is linearly proportional to the haematocrit up to nearly 30% and that the slope 0.074 reflects the influence of red cells on P_i/P_0. Next slide (Fig. 3.8). If we increase the haematocrit to above 30%, then the

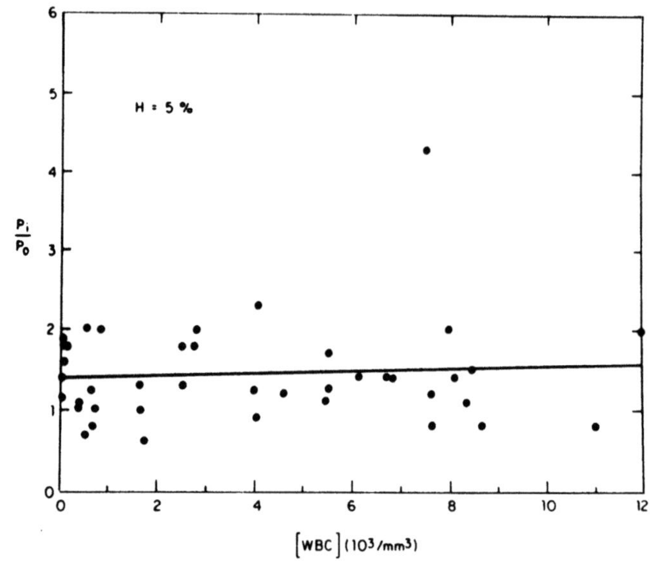
H = 5 %
$\frac{P_i}{P_0}$
[WBC] (10^3/mm^3)

Fig. 3.6

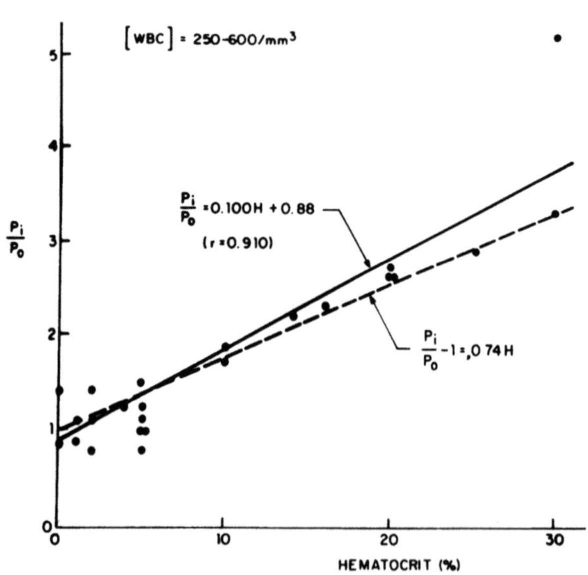
[WBC] = 250-600/mm^3
$\frac{P_i}{P_0}$ = 0.100H + 0.88
(r = 0.910)
$\frac{P_i}{P_0}$ - 1 = 0.74H
$\frac{P_i}{P_0}$
HEMATOCRIT (%)

Fig. 3.7

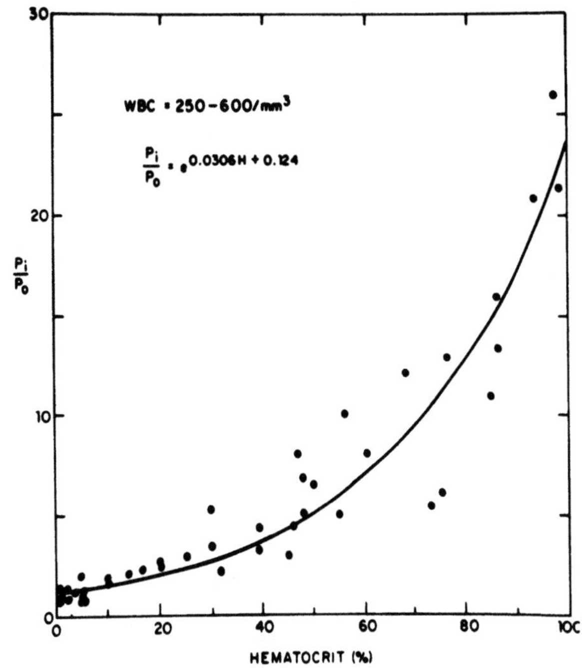

Fig. 3.8

relationship becomes curvilinear. As Dr Skalak pointed out, in our theory we assume only one cell per pore at any given time. At such high haematocrits there are probably multiple cells in each pore, and hence the relationship departs from the linearity seen for haematocrit up to about 25%.

In the next slide (Fig. 3.9) the parameter k_1 is the slope of the earlier rapid rise of the pressure (after the P_i has been obtained) divided by P_0. On this slide k_1 is plotted against the white cell concentration, which is given in number of WBC per mm^3 on the lower abscissa and in leukocrit (H*, volume percent of WBC) on the upper abscissa. At a constant haematocrit of 5%, variations in white cell concentration have a strong influence on k_1; k_1 and [WBC] are positively correlated with a coefficient of correlation of 0.75. It is to be noted that, even at [WBC] of 10,000/mm^3, the leukocrit is still very low (only 0.2%). This supports what Dick Skalak said earlier that a 2% leukocrit is already quite high. Slide (Fig. 3.10). The value of k_1 is a function of not only the white cell concentration but also the red cell concentration. When we hold the white cell concentration within a narrow range while varying the red cell concentration, k_1 can be shown to be correlated with the haematocrit (lower abscissa) or red cell concentration (upper abscissa). Therefore, k_1 is correlated with both the red cell and the white cell concentrations.

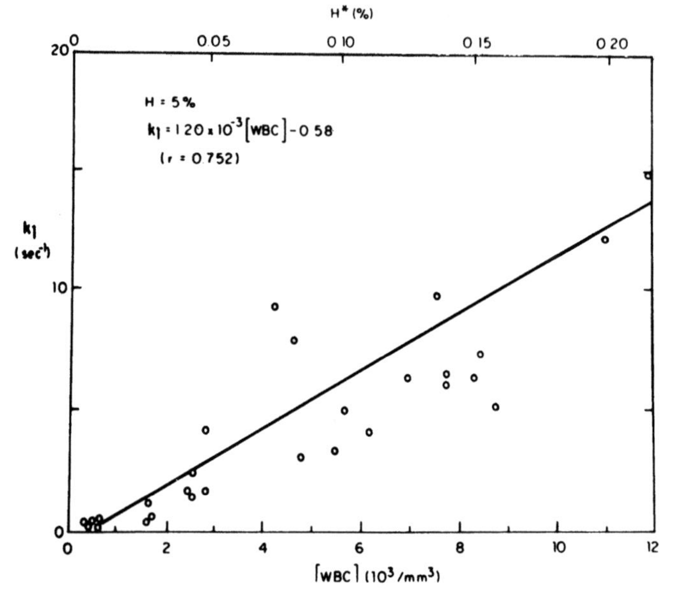

Fig. 3.9

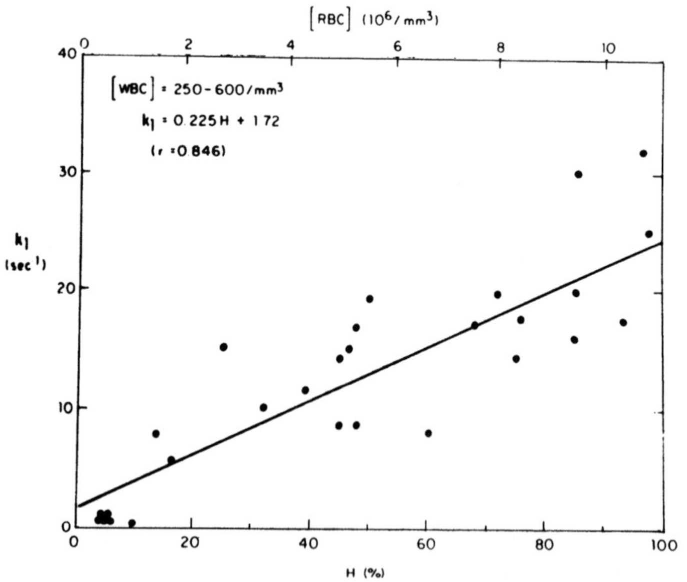

Fig. 3.10

Slide (Fig. 3.11). These data are combined on this slide where k_1 is plotted against the number concentration of cells per mm^3 (bottom abscissa for both the red cell and the white cell). The top abscissa is the volume concentration (the haematocrit or the leukocrit). The scales for the two types of cells are not exactly superimposed because of the difference in mean corpuscular volume, which is approximately twice as big for the white cell as compared to the red cell; therefore there is a displacement of the top abscissa by a factor of 2. In order to get a given k_1 value, the red cell concentration needed is about 3 orders of magnitude higher than the white cell concentration, i.e. you need 1,000 times as many red cells as the white cells to cause the same rate of pressure rise in the earlier rapid phase.

Slide (Fig. 3.12). Similarly, a plot of the slope k_2 for the later, slower phase of pressure rise against the cell concentration also shows that the curve for the white cell is displaced to the right as compared with that for the red cell by about 3 orders of magnitude, i.e. with a ratio of about 1,000 to 1. It is interesting to note that the red cell concentration in normal blood is approximately 3 orders of magnitude higher than the white cell concentration. Furthermore, the viscosity of the haemoglobin solution inside the red cell with a normal MCHC is less than 0.1 poise, and our micropipette studies on individual white cells yield a viscosity value of close to 100 poises; thus the viscosity parameters of these two types of cell also differ by 3 orders of magnitude.

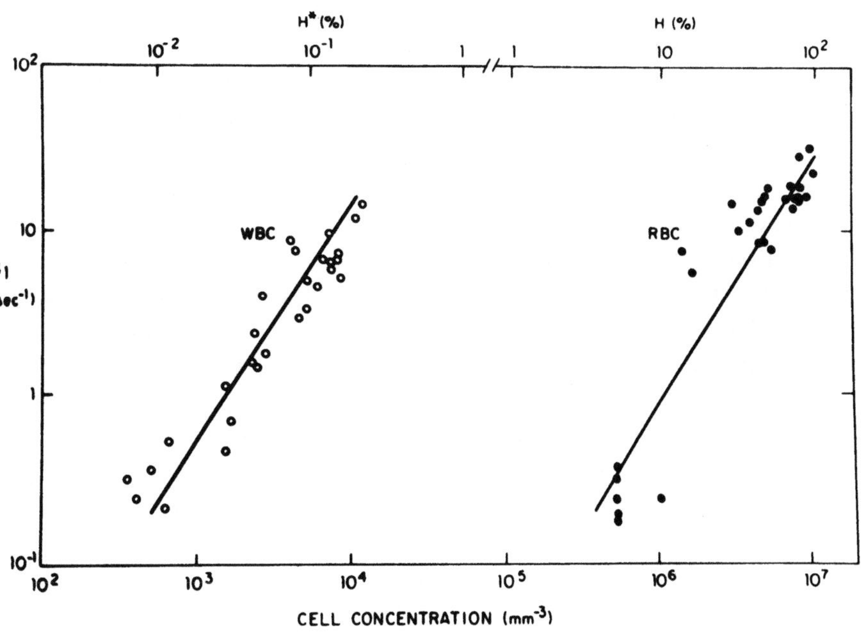

Fig. 3.11

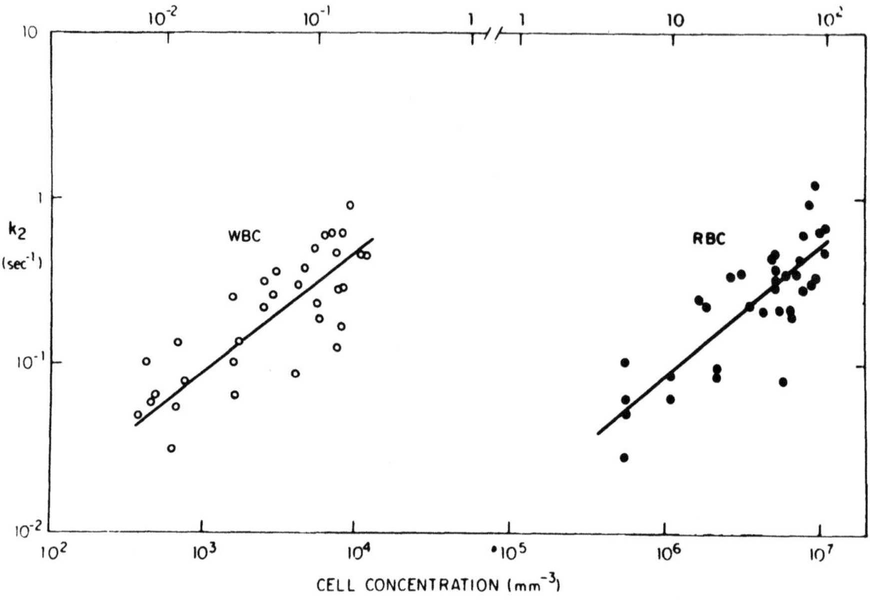

Fig. 3.12

Slide (Fig. 3.13). The results have been analysed by using the theory presented by Dick Skalak. The theoretical modelling includes the plugging of pores during filtration, and some of the pores are assumed to be permanently plugged, probably mainly by the white cells. This transmission electron micrograph taken from a filter following filtration test with a relatively high concentration of white cells shows the filter pores plugged by white cells. The plugging involves mainly the granulocytes; there are very few lymphocytes or monocytes caught in the pores. Slide (Fig. 3.14). Scanning electron microscopic examination of the downstream side of the filter has demonstrated the formation of bouquets of cells attached (or adhered) to the filter pore near the exit. In this picture the bouquet contains one white cell (ruffled surface), which was probably the first cell to be caught, and the red cells (the other cells with smooth surfaces) were then trapped subsequently.

Slide (Fig. 3.15). The solid line in the slide shows the experimental data on the filtration pressure P normalised for P_0 plotted against time. At 0 time, the filtration flow begins, and the pressure jumps up to the P_i value and then rises further with time over the 80-second period of recording. The wavy nature of the experimental curve is probably due to the imperfect nature of the pump. By choosing parameters such as β for the red cell, the corresponding β^* value for the white cell and using the known values of the feed haematocrit (H_f) and leukocrit ($H_f{}^*$), we can fit the experimental curve with the theory that Dick Skalak discussed. In this fitting procedure, we can vary the percentages of the entering red cells or white cells which will plug the pores transiently (E and E* respectively), or permanently (E_p and E_p*, respectively) as well as the rate of cell unplugging (E_u). The results indicate that the experimental data can be fitted reasonably well by the theory, although for some curves the fitting is not as good as shown here. With the improvement of the theory by introducing the distribution function that Dick Skalak mentioned, we probably can get an even better fitting. The results of the fitting of several experimental curves give the following parameters for normal blood cells. The percent of the entering white cells that cause transient plugging (E*) is about 65%, i.e. two thirds of the white cells will get held up in the filter. In this modelling procedure, E for red cells is taken to be 1/700 of E* because the ratio of the relative effectiveness of these two types of cells in causing k_1 to increase is about 1:700. The transiently trapped cells are unplugged at a rate (E_u) of approximately 4% per sec per unit pressure rise. Approximately 2% of the entering white cells will get permanently lodged (E_p*) in the filter, whereas E_p for red cells is taken to be 1/1000 of E_p*. In the new modelling approach using a distribution function that Dick Skalak mentioned, this 'permanent' plugging is attributable to those white cells with extremely slow

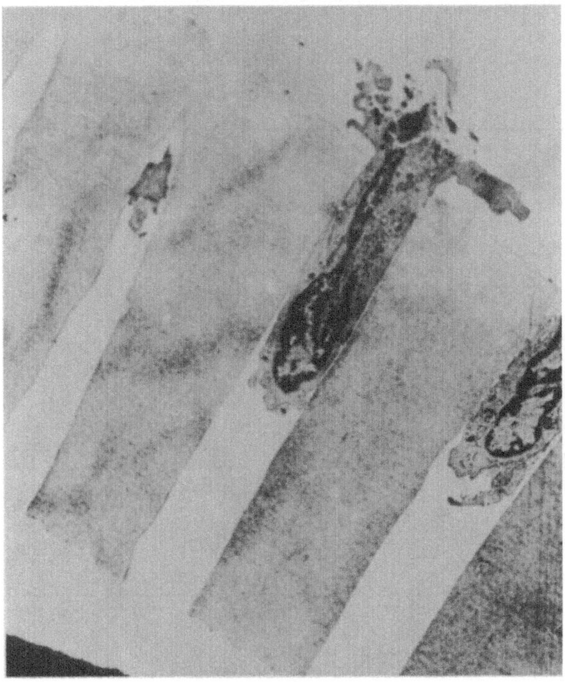

Fig. 3.13

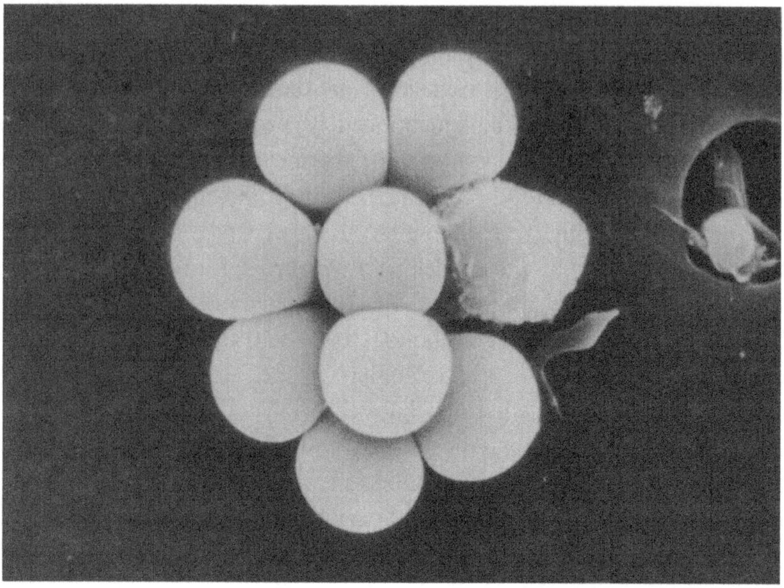

Fig. 3.14

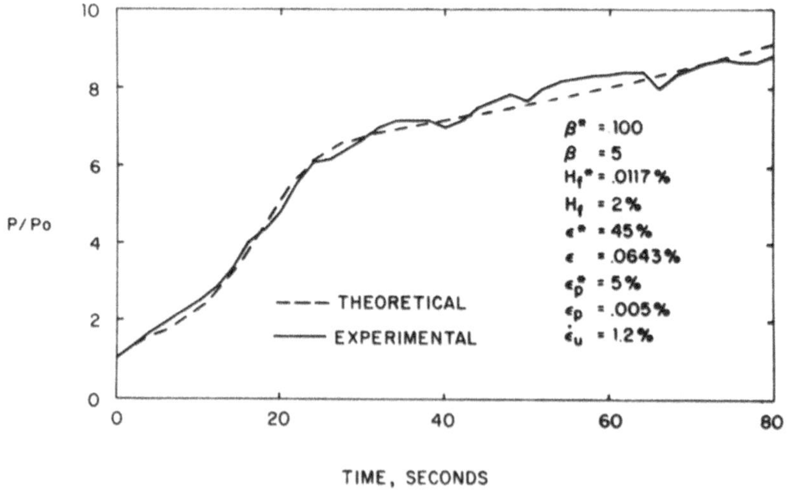

Fig. 3.15

transit time. In summary, by analysing the filtration pressure–time curves obtained with various feed haematocrits and leukocrits, we can derive some parameters such as the deformability of the red cell (β), the deformability of the white cell (β^*), the percent of those cells that will get held up in the pores transiently (E and E*) and permanently (E_p and E_p*), and the rate at which the cells get unplugged (E_u). These analyses are still preliminary, and we are in the process of improving them. The purpose of these investigations is to understand the microrheological basis of each component of the filtration curve under normal conditions and to establish the basis for interpreting abnormal results in filtration tests in disease.

Slide (Fig. 3.16). Knowing the β value for the red cells, we can calculate the fraction (α) of the pores occupied by the red cell. In the equation shown on the slide, h is the fractional volume concentration of red cell, or feed haematocrit/100 and V is the volume ratio of a red cell to a pore. As pointed out earlier by Dick Skalak, at a feed haematocrit of 10% you could have as much as 60% of the pores occupied by the red cells; with a feed haematocrit of 30%, almost every pore has a red cell. The reason for these high values of α is because of the slower rate of transit of the red cell as compared to the suspending fluid. At 0 time, when the filtration flow begins, the cell concentration in the pore is the same as that in the feed suspension. But soon after that, because the red cells go more slowly than

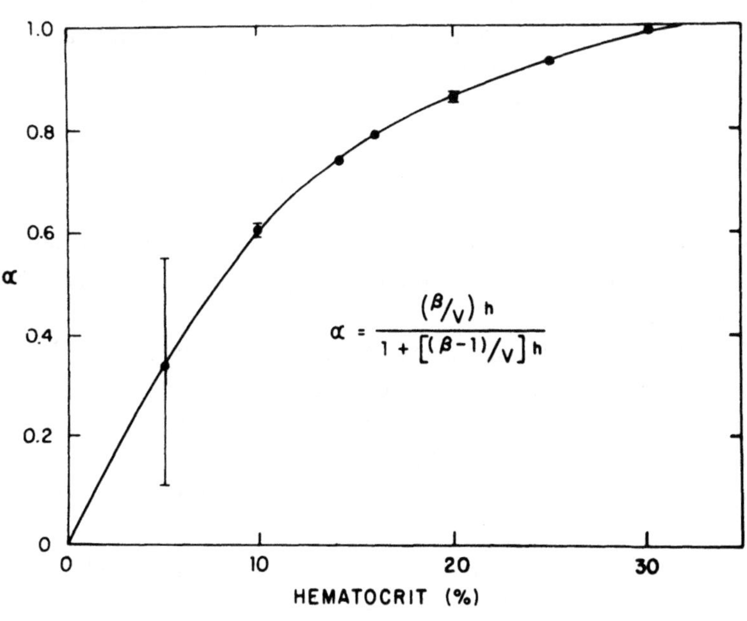

Fig. 3.16

the suspending fluid, there are a lot more red cells in the filter than in the approaching flow. The white cells are not important in the beginning when you suddenly bring up the flow, because of their usually low feed concentration. But if you allow time to proceed, then the very slow transit time of white cells amplifies their number in the filter. If we were able to freeze the filter momentarily, we would see that most of the pores are occupied by the white cells, even though they exist in very small concentration in the approaching flow. Thank you very much.

P.G. I think we should have comments and questions to both sessions. I see all hands up.

J.S. If 1000 red cells do the job of one white cell and normal blood has 1000 more red cells than white cells, then in bulk the white cell contribution from normal blood has the same effect as the red cell contribution.

S.C. Yes, I would think so, at least for 5 μm vessels. This refers to relatively long periods of filtration. The P_i is less affected by the smaller number of white cells.

J.S. So, if you assume now a 6 minute pumping time as in many systems, how many white cells would you have to remove before you would accept that the system was measuring red cell filtration? Do you have to be less that 1% white cells left?

S.C. Because of the strong amplification effect I mentioned before, even 1% white cells could have a significant effect. If β^* equals 1000, that means each white cell will traverse the filter pore 1000 times slower than the buffer. So each white cell in the feed is equivalent to a lot more in the pore. But to answer your question regarding the quantitative effect at 6 minutes, we have to do some calculation using the theory.

R.S. I always say look at the data. Don't you have a slide that shows at some very low white cell concentration what the rise is? I think that would be interesting.

J.S. To restate the question, should we all abandon long pumping times or can we still retain a 6 minute pumping time providing we remove, let's say, 99% of the white cells reliably?

S.C. One can pump as long as one wants, but we should not look at just one number, instead we should look at the curve, from which we can derive the P_i and the slope rise. Of course, the later part of the pumping may generate a pressure so high that you get haemolysis and other problems.

J.S. So for several reasons you should not pump for many minutes. We are pumping too long.

S.C. That is right. I think the later part is not very valuable. The shorter the better. I do not think you need 6 minutes.

J.S. Your data applied to heparinised blood, how many hours after venipuncture were the experiments done?

S.C. These studies were performed from volunteers in the lab, so they were done within 2 hours.

J.S. Do you think heparin has an effect on leukocyte aggregation above the filter?

S.C. Yes, heparin would cause more aggregation of white cells than EDTA.

J.S. This may increase the number of white cells in your filter holder by causing aggregation on the surface of the filter and accentuating the effects.

S.C. If you aggregate the white cells certainly it would accentuate the filter plugging, because each clump of white cells is bigger than the individual white cells. Dick Skalak wanted me to use the experiment to answer John Stuart's question. Slide 1 does not cover a sufficient range of white cell concentration. We should use plots showing a wide range of white cell concentrations.

R.S. But the bottom left hand curve in slide 3.5 gives one point of data of interest to the question. He has 10 white cells and the pressure is still rising. What is the length of time there?

S.C. This curve lasts approximately 1 minute.

R.S. OK, so if he goes on for 6 minutes, it is still going to go up when there are only 10 white cells per mm^3. That is what I wanted to see, the data is really striking.

S.C. The effect is there, and it is a function of time. But the 5% haematocrit in this suspension may be the main reason of the plugging in this curve.

P.L. In the system we use we have made a few very basic simplistic assumptions. You start from the assumption that normal whole blood has a haematocrit of 45% with 5 million red blood cells per mm^3, and 5,000 white blood cells indiscriminate of the type of white blood cells. It is also assumed that 1 white blood cell can occlude 1 pore; that is very simplistic from what we have heard. The usual 5 micron 13 mm Nuclepore disc likely has 3×10^5 available pores once it is mounted, and we will leave aside the 3 micron filters that I use. By removing the buffy coat we find the best one can do is reduce the white cell concentration by a factor of 5. The only other way you have to reduce the number of white cells in relation to the number of pores is to dilute the whole suspension, and that is the main reason why we have been working at such low haematocrits as 0.01%, which is 10,000 red blood cells per microlitre. One ml of whole blood at 40% haematocrit without removing the white cells has 5×10^6 white cells; since the filter has only 3×10^5 pores you would obviously block everything with 1 ml of suspension. You can divide it whichever way you want. If you remove the white cells by washing, you still end up with 8.8×10^5 white cells per ml, that is still more than 200% the number of pores you have available. If you dilute down to 5% haematocrit, then you have 36% of your pores in a 5 micron filter that will be clogged after 1 ml of suspension. In the systems that you read in the literature, people usually filter more than 1 ml. If you go down to 1% haematocrit, then you have 7% of your pores occluded, and you can keep on diluting. In terms of numbers it gives you an idea, based on that very simple assumption that one white cell blocks one pore, how much you really have to remove white cells if you do not want to get into any significant problems.

H.M. Shu, I'd like to ask about the last slide you showed and then the earlier ones where you are computing basically k_1 and k_2. The place where the data was the worst, or the scatter is the largest, of the last slide where α was calculated from the β was at the lowest haematocrits.

S.C. Yes.

H.M. Things look much better above 10 or 15% haematocrit.

S.C. Yes, that is correct.

H.M. What does that mean?

S.C. I think that is a very good point, I meant to bring it up but I did not. At low haematocrits P_i is very close to P_0; therefore when you calculate the β from $P_i - P_0/P_0$ you are dealing with a very tiny difference. The error due to any inaccuracy in the pressure measurement is thus magnified. At very low pressures, e.g. 1 mm Hg or so, the measurement error is very large. Since you use the β to calculate the α, the error is carried through to the α value. This therefore suggests that in performing the filtration tests we should not go to too low a haematocrit. The choice of the haematocrit is sort of a compromise. Pierre pointed out that if you use a high haematocrit you have a concurrently high leukocyte concentration, which you want to get down by diluting the suspension. But if you dilute it too much, you don't have enough red cells to work with and the error becomes greater.

H.M. In your last slide, when you calculated the α knowing the β, at the lowest haematocrit you had a large standard deviation and all of a sudden the data become collapsed at higher haematocrits.

S.C. That is right.

H.M. So you are saying 20% or higher would be better.

S.C. In the papers in press in *Biorheology*, we recommend anywhere between 10 and 20% haematocrit. If you go too high then it departs from the assumption that only one cell goes into a pore. So the best is to keep it between 10 and 20% so you get a good pressure to measure with and I think other people, e.g. Holger, also recommended 10%.

P.L. It depends what kind of filter you use. If you lower the number of pores then you can lower the number of cells.

S.C. Yes, of course. You are absolutely right. All we are saying is based on the particular filter we used.

M.H. I do not see the use of your long filtration times. That is very bad. You have got plugging and you do not know what is plugging. It is very complicated and there is another complication which you probably have not taken into account. It is the concentration of red blood cells just in front of the membrane which is increasing all the time so that at the end of your 6 minutes the red blood cells have got to go through a highly concentrated region just before the membrane and then you have a multi-filtration system and you do not know what you are doing.

S.C. I agree with you that there is no point in pumping for a long time. The point is that you look at time history of the curve and want to know what is the basis for each part. Our results indicate that P_i represents the properties of the red cells and the later parts represent mainly the plugging of the pores by white cells.

M.H. Yes, the idea is to use as low as possible haematocrit and make the measurement as fast as possible. I have another question. It is the Gregersen and Bryant paper a long time ago. I think I remember that the transit time at the beginning was much longer than the one you calculated. Is that correct? I think that in paper it was in the few seconds region.

S.C. It is in the book on Haemorheology edited by Dr Copley (1968).

R.S. Is there a time of transit in there?

M.H. Yes, there is a curve if I remember. Another question or comment was that I thought we did not do a very good job by only decreasing the white blood cell count by a factor of 9, but I think that is a good figure. Shall we speak about the white blood cell fractionation or not?

P.G. If you can make it very short we can, but it would have to be very short.

M.H. How to take the white cells out? The usual technique is to take the buffy coat out and resuspend all the red blood cells. In doing this you resuspend also all the aggregates which are at the bottom of the tube and then you have got to wash it again; it is a long procedure. We use a procedure where we just take a small sample of the red blood cells in the middle of the tube. So it is much faster, and I think the white blood cell exclusion is higher than in the normal technique. There could be some selection of red blood cells, but this is not the case because in the usual centrifugation technique the discrimination between young and old cells is very low, as shown by other people. We do not get the reticulocytes, of course, but we are not interested in that, so we do not need to have them.

G.L. Question to Holger. Has he put Professor Hanss' selected population of red cells from the middle of the packed red cell column through the SER, because I suspect you may be losing that population of abnormal red cells skewed to the right which I believe we are going to be interested in looking at, are we not?

H.S.-S. This is possible. We were so much involved in this anticoagulant business that we have not had a chance to look at the distribution by selecting them on the basis of specific gravity, so this is up as one of the next projects.

P.G. I think we should now move on. You had a comment?

H.S.-S. One comment and one question. L. Heilmann of Essen, who is interested in the rheology of neonatal blood and pregnant women, has attempted what you have done, namely to measure the pressure with a constant flow system and he eventually gave up. So in the clinical setting with whole blood I would just like to have your comment on that, it is impossible to get any reproducible curve, they are jerky, erratic. Even if we were to go back and look at these records, I do not think even the initial part is anything close to your curves which you have in very highly purified systems, if I am correct. In other words, do you have any experience with this sort of analysis in the real life lab situation?

S.C. The problem really lies in the sample rather than in the approach. I think if you use whole blood there are certain problems in there that can cause variability, the degree of red cell aggregation or platelet aggregation, white cell sticking and so forth, and it will not be reproducible no matter what instrument you use. I would think that if a sample is not reproducible in terms of initial pressure on a constant flow, you will also have a problem with initial flow at constant pressure. At 0 time those two measurements are related to each other. Of course, each instrument must be able to reproduce results for a purified cell suspension with a small error range. If both the pressure measurement and the flow measurement are sufficiently accurate, then the two methods should give the same result at 0 time. Subsequently they give different results; in one case the pressure will rise and in the other case the flow will go down.

P.G. John Dormandy will now present his analysis.

J.D. I would like to present some experimental data on the effect of white cells and a slightly different analysis of results, which is very simple and therefore possibly wrong. We used the mark 2 technique of red cell filterability which involves a 5% suspension of red cells in the plasma after removing the buffy coat. At first sight it would seem that if the white cell count in the suspension is less than 0.2×10^9, then it does not seem to make too much difference to the filtration rate. But as soon as the white cell count gets higher, which it does in fact in many cases, then it will significantly interfere with the apparent red cell filterability. But on closer examination, even below a concentration of 0.2×10^9 the white cell count matters. In this table we have simply divided the white cell count in the suspension into three groups, all below 0.2×10^9. We then looked at

WBC suspension (10^9/l)	<0.05	0.05–0.15	>0.15	r
WBC in original blood (10^9/l)	7.8	7.7	7.7	NS
RCF (ml/min)	0.54	0.51	0.47	P<0.01
Plasma viscosity (mPas)	1.26	1.31	1.35	P<0.01
Red cell count (10^{12}/l)	0.54	0.52	0.53	NS
Haemoglobin (g/dl)	1.8	1.8	1.8	NS
Mean red cell volume (fl)	88	89	90	NS
MCHC (g/dl)	39	40	39	NS
n	22	25	8	

r: Coefficient of rank correlation

Fig. 3.17

these variables in the three groups. (The samples came from both normals and patients.) The only correlation we could find was with filtration time and the plasma viscosity. Therefore, even at this low concentration the white cells affect filtration time. The correlation between the plasma viscosity and the number of white cells in suspension might possibly be related to the plasma viscosity, or the proteins in the plasma, altering the proportion of the white cells remaining in the centrifuged red cells. There is no correlation at all between the number of white cells in the suspension and the white cells in the original blood. So filtration tests are not simply measuring the white cells in the patient, but rather the tendency of the white cells to be removed from the red cells by centrifugation. We tried to analyse the result we get slightly differently and I would like to advocate the merits of a constant pressure, or more or less constant pressure system and go back to what we decided last year. If you had no clogging at all, then if you plot the filtration rate against the volume filtered there would be no problem because the filtration rate would be constant. If there is clogging then you would get this line which would have a constant slope assuming that the concentration of clogging particles remains the same and therefore a certain volume going through the filter will always contain the same number of clogging particles. And

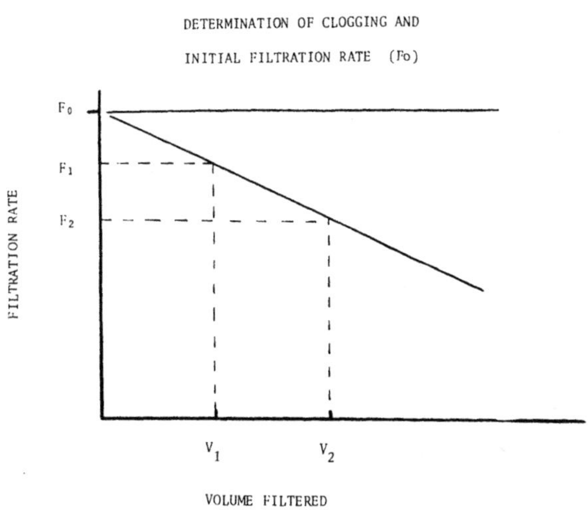

$$Fo = \frac{F_1(V_2/V_1)-F_2}{V_2/V_1-1}$$

$$C = N(F_0-F_1)/F_0/V_1$$

C : Blocking particles per ml

N : Number of pores in the filter

Fig. 3.18

if you accept that this line is straight, then theoretically you could extrapolate back to F_0, which is the filtration rate at the very beginning, in the absence of clogging. All you need to do to achieve this is to measure the filtration rates (F_1 and F_2) after filtering two known volumes of blood (V_1 and V_2). Theoretically it should not matter where these two points are, all you have to know is the filtration rate at two points in time and the volume filtered at those points. You can then simply extrapolate back and get F_0. The slide shows the appropriate formula to use. F_0 ought to be the filtration rate in the absence of clogging particles and the concentration of blocking particles (c) can also be calculated. This slide (Fig. 3.19) summarises the many reasons why I think we ought to use a constant pressure system rather than a constant flow system. Again, in the top half the filtration rate is plotted against the volume filtered. In the lower half the filtration pressure is plotted against volume filtered. Now the top represents a constant pressure system where you will have a constant flow rate of the suspension medium, a constant red cell transit time and a constant clogging rate. In a constant flow system where the pressure varies we have just heard that you get a variable clogging rate because as the pressure rises some of the blocked pores

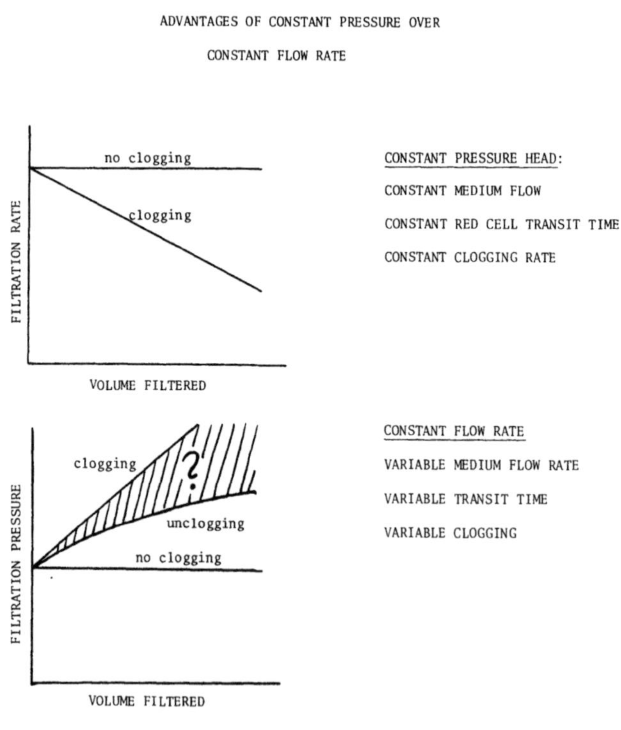

Fig. 3.19

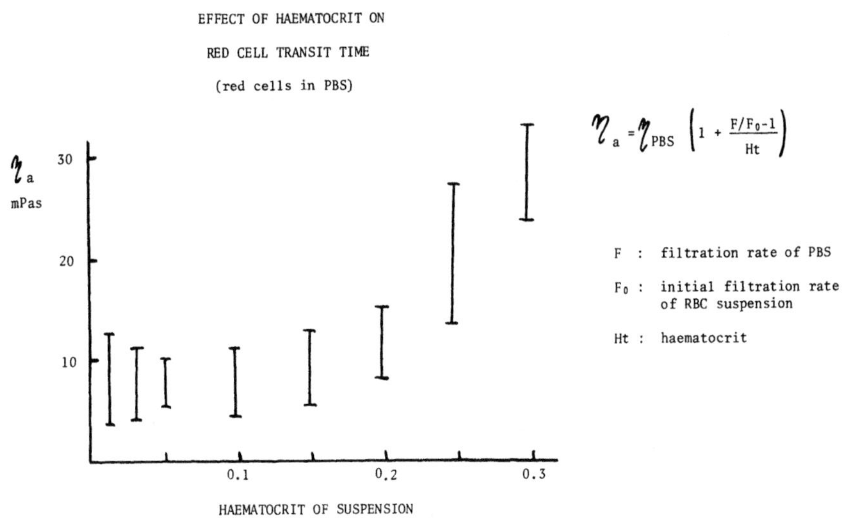

Fig. 3.20

become unblocked. So instead of a straight line, you get a curve depending on the amount of unblocking. Furthermore, there will be a variable rate of medium flow as the pressure rises as well as a variable rate of clogging. This morning we also heard that at higher pressures you might also get haemolysis. So I would argue the merits of a constant pressure system rather than a constant flow system.

My last slide (Fig. 3.20) shows the effect of the haematocrit on the red cell transit time. F_0 is the calculated transit time or filtration rate at zero point in time in the absence of clogging, obtained by extrapolation as shown before. And that is plotted here against the haematocrit. There is no significant change in the initial filtration rate up to haematocrit, or a packed cell volume, of about 0.15. So as far as haematocrit goes, it would seem that somewhere in the range of 10% to 15% is reasonable. Thank you.

P.G. Questions and comments on this presentation?

G.L. I think you must get unclogging also in the constant pressure system. If you are progressively blocking the pores you are reducing the total surface area of holes across your membrane. Is that not going to result in some build-up of pressure above each pore area?

J.D. The pressure above the hole is going to depend on hydrostatic pressure of the fluid above it. It does not matter whether it is one hole or 1,000.

P.L. But it will affect the flow rate, though, all the time.

J.D. It will affect the flow rate, but linearly against the volume filtered. But the pressure changes hardly at all. The more we hear about the analysis of pressure curves, the more convinced I get that a constant pressure system is probably better.

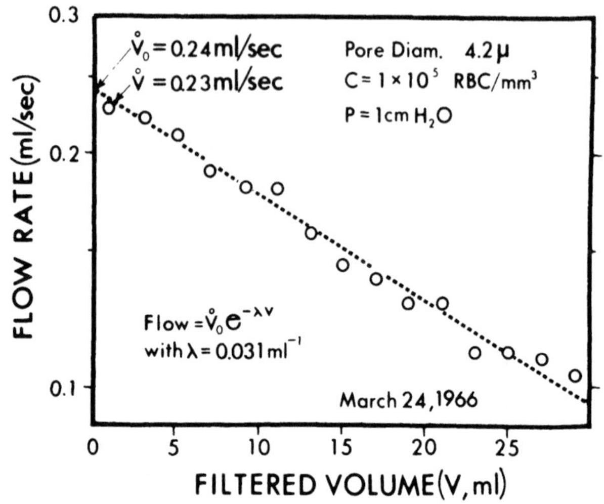

Fig. 3.21

S.C. This slide (Fig. 3.21) actually presages the previous presentation and dates back to 1966 when we did use a constant pressure and measured the flow. Indeed, we used this extrapolation technique with Professor Gregersen, and you get a 0 time flow out of this. The extrapolated flow value approximates initial flow, i.e. the very first point, just as Dr Hanss is doing. So I think you can either extrapolate or take the very early reading, which would do the job.

J.D. Why was it abandoned?

S.C. It was not abandoned. The constant pressure and constant flow methods are the same if you go to the 0 time. The question is the ease of doing the pressure or the flow measurement. Now Dr Hanss has the instrument and makes it a lot easier to measure flow, but in those days to measure the flow was more difficult than to measure the pressure. It is a matter of convenience rather than anything else.

J.D. With a constant pressure system it does not matter where you make the measurements as you are working on a straight line. Theoretically you can make your measurements wherever you want to.

S.C. Normally I think they probably are like this. In abnormal situations are you sure that there will always be a semi-logarithmic exponential decay?

J.D. Of course Professor Hanss' machine would have to be adapted slightly because you do need two points. So you need to know the flow rate at two points in time but his machine currently can only read at one point.

S.C. I think it all depends on what you are looking for. If you want the red cell deformability you want the initial resistance, then I think it does not matter which approach you use to get it. The problem arises in the later phase. The initial readings should be the same, whether you use the constant pressure or the constant flow.

P.G. Thank you very much. I think we still keep within the framework of this topic and now Peter Buchan is next on the programme.

P.B. Slide (Fig. 3.12). I am glad that I used a constant pressure system after following John's presentation. This is based on his setup and what I was doing here was measuring in whole blood, over 20 second periods, the volume progressively filtered. So it is the same filter, filter for 20 seconds, measure the volume, measure the volume, measure the volume and so we see a progressive clogging effect. Which is just what John illustrated before. Slide (Fig. 3.23). And this is looking up again at one of these filters seeing these little grapes, or

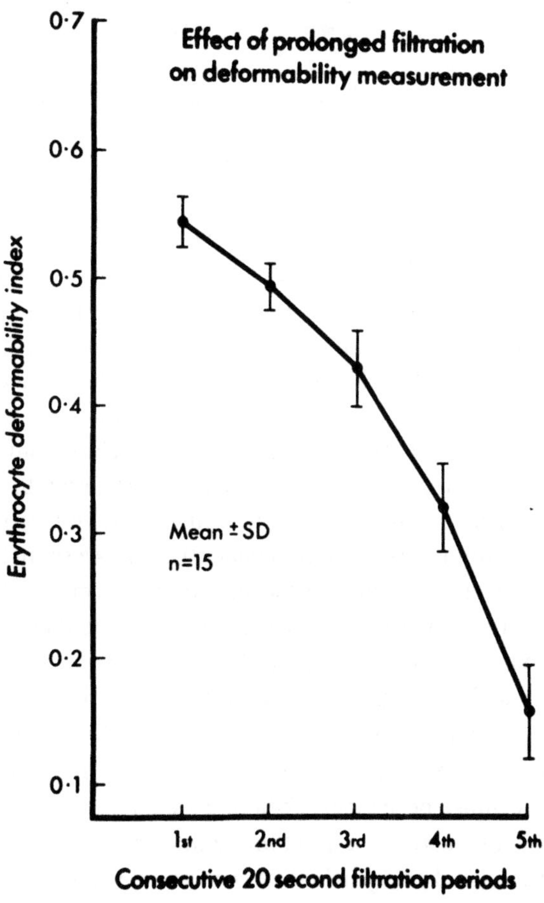

Fig. 3.22

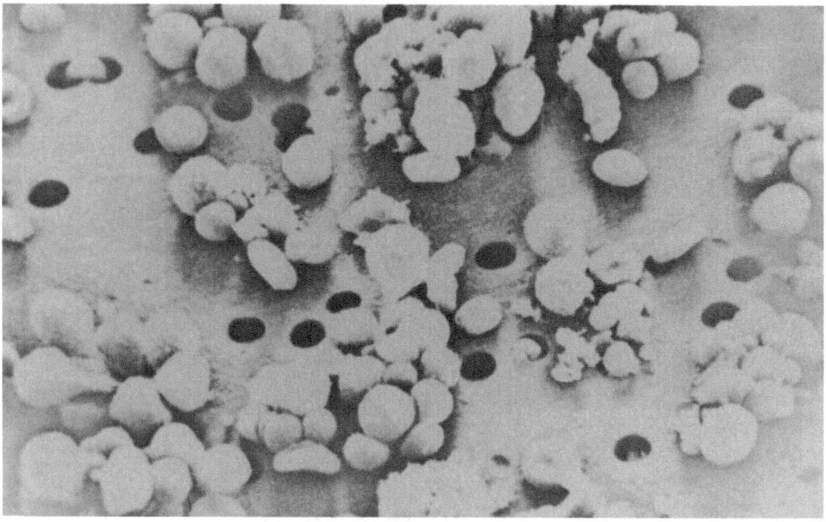

Fig. 3.23

whatever. This is largely made up of white cells. Slide (Fig. 3.24). The close-up shows many of these cells, largely white cells, coming through and being caught up. It appeared to me that in the subjects I was looking at who physiologically had a high white count, that is in the neonate and in pregnancy, they have almost double the sort of average adult white count, that there may be something different. In my adult female patients, pregnant women, patients who had a post-operative infection (in my practice that is very seldom but it occasionally happens) and babies in the first week of life, I looked at the white cell count in the blood I was putting in and in the filtrate after filtering for 60 seconds with whole blood (Fig. 3.25). I found that in adult females there was a small fall-off in white blood cells after filtration, in pregnant women there was more fall-off, and most in the post-operative patients. By contrast in the neonate there was only a very small fall-off. So it was not just a matter of the number of white cells presenting itself to the filters. There was something different in these two situations, it appeared to me, that may account for this increased stickiness of the white blood cells. I then did electromicrographs of the pores of the filters I was using and looked at the percentage pore blockage taking a standard area of the pore under the scanning electron microscope and I found that again with adult females 20% of the pores were blocked by white cells after one minute of whole blood filtration, in the pregnant group 40%, in the post-op 50%, and in the neonate only 15%. And I would be interested to hear what people think about this, as to

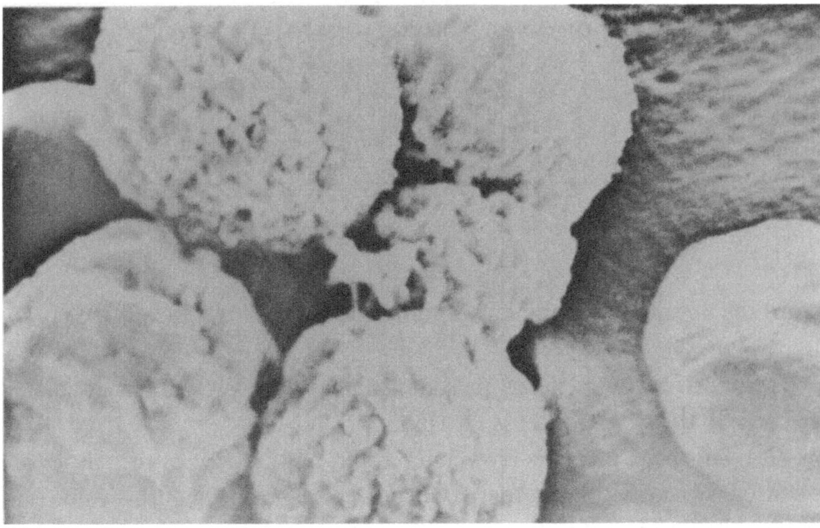

Fig. 3.24

whether for instance this is an effect of plasma proteins which are elevated in pregnancy and post-operatively. This is an observation of the importance of removing white blood cells and what they can do if we do not remove them. Thank you.

P.G. I noticed that Pierre's hand was up before Peter was actually finished.

P.L. As a haematologist, it seems to me that it goes along well with the various proportions of granulocytes to lymphocytes that you see in the blood of these different individuals. It seems fairly clear to me that you lose more cells in situations where the proportion of granulocytes in the blood is larger. You do not lose very many in the neonates because they have more lymphocytes. You lose a lot in post-operative infection because this is mostly granulocytes. This morning we heard about temperature effects, and I would like all of you to think of what temperature does to granulocytes. For example, I am sure there may be quite a bit of what we see of temperature effects especially in whole blood experiments that is due to granulocytes sticking or not sticking. A granulocyte at 4° is round and a granulocyte at 37° is flat and sticky.

P.G. Further questions or comments?

S.C. I agree with what Pierre has said. When we examine the filter we only see the granulocytes plugging the pore. Furthermore, the computed plugging percentage of the white cells turns out to be about some 60%, which is also the percentage of granulocytes in the white cell population. So both of these will

	WBC	
	Before	After
Adult women	7.4	7.1
Pregnant	11.6	10.2
Post-operative	16.8	12.5
Neonate	14.5	13.8

Fig. 3.25

support the notion that granulocytes rather than lymphocytes cause filter plugging.

P.G. No further comments or questions to this point? We will come back to it, I am sure. So the next speaker is Dr Hanss.

M.H. I will speak a couple of minutes about haematocrit of the suspension. We started with an 8% haematocrit. Of course, the precision of this value is not very high; it is difficult to measure 8% haematocrit. You cannot do it with the Coulter machine because as you know the result depends on the deformability. So we used a conductivity method to measure this 8% haematocrit with a better precision than the usual microcentrifuge technique. Then the suspensions with lower haematocrits were diluted from the 8%. The filtration index, which has been corrected for haematocrit, was constant at these different haematocrit levels. Those results indicate that the filtration index is an intrinsic red blood cell property and does not depend on the interaction between the cells. From this we can calculate the transit time and we have the same figure as the single erythrocyte rigidometer. Thank you.

P.G. Questions or immediate comments to this presentation? We will stay with the topic of haematocrit, I am sure.

H.S-S. I find this fascinating and there is just one suggestion I would like to make. Could you just simply take the inverse of this? Because you are measuring the volume at given times it would be much easier if your filtration index went up as the cells deteriorate. So why don't you just simply invert this whole thing and then you have relative flow rate corrected for haematocrit.

G.A.M. In our laboratory we have a solution. We don't call it a filtration index anymore, we call it a Hanss index.

H.S.-S. OK, so we should talk about the inverted Hanss index.

M.H. I have thought about doing it the other way around, but it is complicated because then when the cell is very pliable the figures would be very, very high.

P.L. Just a short comment about the difficulties of measuring an 8% haematocrit. Why do we not talk about so many cells per mm^3? Is is much easier to count cells with counters and then dilute them to a particular fraction.

H.M. I recall last year one of the reasons for this haematocrit session was the comment that I think Dick made which was, why don't we do what protein chemists do, or suspension rheologists do, and extrapolate back to 0 haematocrit?

S.C. Both Dr Hanss' and my presentation give you that answer. I mean his IF index and our beta value are like an intrinsic viscosity value. I think John Dormandy also showed that in his last slide. The beta value is obtained by taking the relative pressure reading (P_i/P_0) minus 1, and then dividing that by the red cell count or haematocrit. That is the beta. So that is the resistance offered by each individual cell normalised by the resistance of the suspending medium.

R.S. I think this beta value and Dr Hanss' index are almost one and the same thing. They are close relatives and I promise to do the algebra tonight and bring it back to you tomorrow to see exactly how they correlate.

S.C. I think they are really the same thing. I'd like to return to the point Holger raised earlier regarding the use of time or 1/time. I feel that to use the time is actually good because the time required to filter a given volume is proportionate to the resistance: the higher the resistance, the longer the time. The resistance per cell is what you are after, that is the beta value in our analysis. If you invert it to 1/time, you will be talking about conductance. Of course, you can talk about conductance or resistance, but I think in general we are thinking in terms of resistance more often.

R.S. Shu had a curve where there was a slope of the linear regression of P_i/P_0 versus haematocrit. The index that Dr Hanss is talking about is the slope.

M.H. Yes, indeed.

J.F.S. The purpose of our investigation was to analyse the flow rate curve as a function of volume and the resistance/volume curve at constant pressure (P) for different erythrocyte suspensions. The experimental apparatus described in Fig. 3.26 was constructed in connexion with the Biotechnical Centre n° 23 of the INSERM in Nancy. The device is formed of three main parts: a tank made up of two chambers, A and B, separated by a nuclepore filter (pore size: 5 μm; pore density: $4.10^5/cm^2$; working surface: 0.64 cm^2; number of pores: $2.5 \cdot 10^5$), a pressure generator connected to chamber A, and a gauge for measuring flow rate through the filter.

With the membrane in position between chambers A and B and cock T_1 turned off, a 5 ml sample volume is introduced into chamber A; owing to surface tension, the liquid will only flow out of chamber A if the pressure on the membrane is above several centimeters of water. When cock T_1 is turned on, an increment of pressure is applied in chamber A, the sample flows through the membrane and the FT gauge measures flow rate. Time- and volume-related flow rate (V') as well as volume-related resistance of filter to flow ($R = P/V'$) are provided simultaneously and continuously by an electronic system.

The pressure generator provides constant pressure that can be adjusted to between 3 and 20 cm of water. Building-up time of the pressure increment in

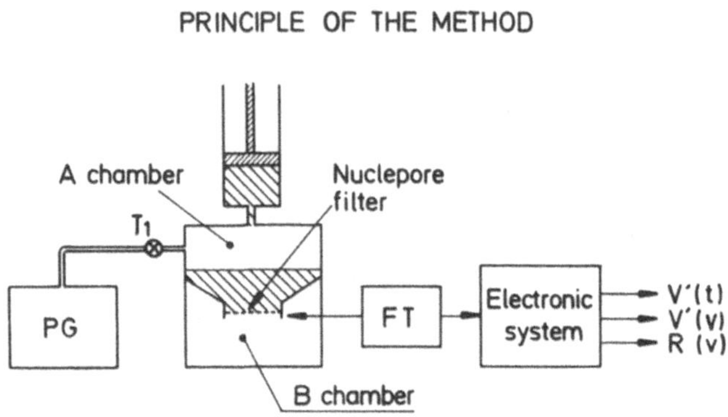

Fig. 3.26

chamber A takes less than 50 ms. Operating time for the flow rate gauge is 20 ms (from 10 to 90% of the final value). For flow rates between 3 μls^{-1} and 166 μls^{-1}, linearity is better than $\pm 3\%$.

Three types of curves were studied: $dV/dt = f(t)_{Pcte}$, $dV/dt = f(V)_{Pcte}$ and $R = f(V)_{Pcte}$.

Two series of experiments were undertaken: one consisted of analyzing the influence of hematocrit on the measurements, the other was for assessing the sensitivity of the method. The influence of hematocrit was studied on normal RBCs, washed twice with a filtered buffer at 5 μm and 0.45 μm (standard buffer + 0.2% albumin). Five different hematocrits were tested: 1%, 2%, 3%, 5% and 10%. On a 5 ml sample volume, and allowing for filter characteristics, the mean number of RBCs per pore was respectively 2.10^3, 4.10^3, 6.10^3, 10^4 and 2.10^4. Test sensitivity was assessed on the basis of a sample that had been prepared using the same buffer as in the preceding test, containing a given number of RBCs per pore (2.10^3) and a variable number of glutaraldehyde treated RBCs. The mean number of treated RBCs per pore varied between 2 and 20 (2, 5, 10 and 20).

Only the $dV/dt = f(V)$ and $R = f(V)$ graphs were analyzed: the $dV/dt = f(t)$ curves are only useful for checking the quality of the manipulation. On account of the dynamics of the recording system (table X4 SEFRAM GMT 101T), make-up time for the flow rate gauge and, possibly, transient phenomena connected with the RBCs (sedimentation), the analyses below are primarily concerned with the data obtained once the phenomenon is established, i.e. approximately 200 ms after pressure has been applied in chamber A.

Fig. 3.27 (a and b) shows the graphs obtained with samples of variable normal RBC concentration. The graphs reveal that the influence of hematocrit is par-

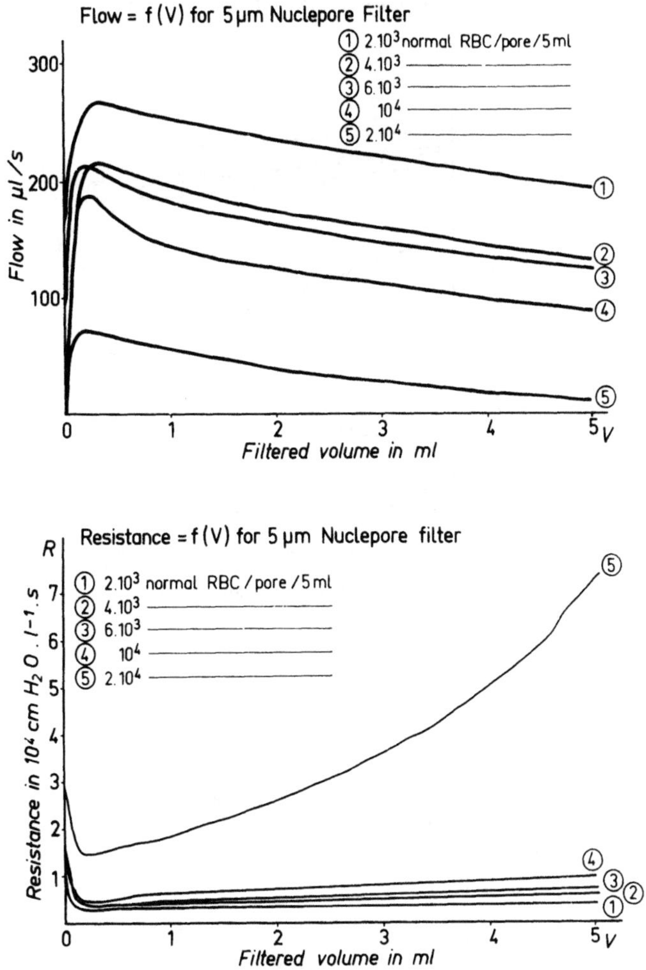

Fig. 3.27

ticularly pronounced when the number of cells flowing through the filter is above 10^4/pore/5 ml. This is shown even more on filter's different resistances to flow according to volume, under the same measuring conditions. A hypothesis can be put forward according to which flow rate is of the quantity $dV/dt = a_1e^{b_1V}$ and resistance $R = a_2e^{b_2V}$. The exponential shape of the graphs is confirmed in Fig. 3.28 (a and b) which represents the same phenomena plotted with a semi-logarithmic scale. Exponential regression carried out on 10 points gives the values a_1, b_1, a_2, b_2, as well as the correlation coefficients and shows that (Fig. 3.29):

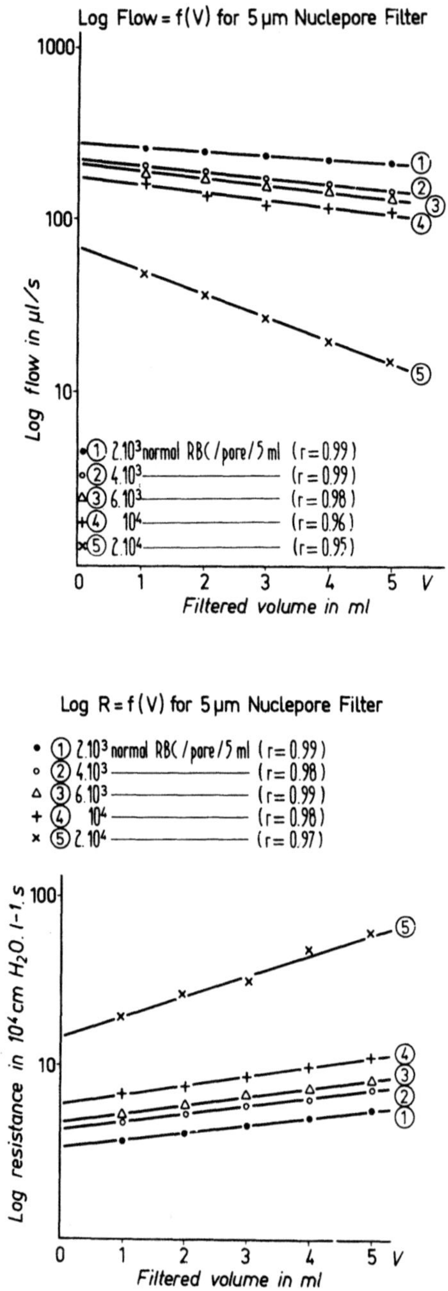

Log Flow = f(V) for 5 μm Nuclepore Filter
1000
100
10
Log flow in μl/s
① 2.10³ normal RBC / pore / 5 ml (r = 0.99)
② 4.10³ (r = 0.99)
③ 6.10³ (r = 0.98)
④ 10⁴ (r = 0.96)
⑤ 2.10⁴ (r = 0.95)
0 1 2 3 4 5 V
Filtered volume in ml
Log R = f (V) for 5 μm Nuclepore Filter
① 2.10³ normal RBC / pore / 5 ml (r = 0.99)
② 4.10³ (r = 0.98)
③ 6.10³ (r = 0.99)
④ 10⁴ (r = 0.98)
⑤ 2.10⁴ (r = 0.97)
100
10
Log resistance in 10⁴ cm H₂O. l-1. s
0 1 2 3 4 5 V
Filtered volume in ml

Fig. 3.28

Exponential regression (N = 10)

$$\frac{dV}{dt} = a_1 e^{b_1 V}$$

Number of normal RBC/pore/5 ml	2.10^3	4.10^3	6.10^3	10^4	2.10^4
R^2	0,99	0,99	0,98	0,96	0,95
a_1	272	233	219	169	66
b_1	−0,07	−0,09	−0,1	−0,14	−0,43

$$\text{Resistance} = a_2 e^{b_2 V}$$

Number of normal RBC/pore/5 ml	2.10^3	4.10^3	6.10^3	10^4	2.10^4
R^2	0,99	0,98	0,99	0,98	0,97
a_2	$3{,}3.10^4$	$4{,}2.10^4$	$4{,}7.10^4$	$5{,}8.10^4$	15.10^4
b_2	0,1	0,12	0,16	0,20	0,33

Fig. 3.29

1) up to the value of 10^4 RBCs/pore/5 ml, the phenomenon can be regarded, fairly approximately, as being exponential,
2) that coefficients a_1 and a_2, which are undoubtedly connected with buffer viscosity, vary according to hematocrit,
3) that coefficients b_1 and b_2, which are very closely connected with hematocrit, could be useful indexes.

When undertaken at low hematocrit, with a and b varying only slightly, the sensitivity tests, the results of which are given in Fig. 3.30 (a and b) clearly illustrate the influence of treated RBCs. Fig. 3.31 (a and b) validate the exponential approach up to 10 treated RBCs/pore/5 ml. Finally, Fig. 3.32, which gives the coefficient values up to 10 treated RBCs/pore/5 ml shows the slight connection between coefficients a and the number of treated RBCs, and confirms the value of coefficients b_1 and b_2, that are connected, in an elementary fashion, to the number hardened-treated RBCs.

Generally good results can be obtained with this technique. Coefficient b_2 connected with the filter's resistance to flow could merely account for RBC filterability. Further tests must be carried out to remove certain minor faults in the system and a study on pathological RBCs is now under consideration.

P.G. Thank you very much. Questions and comments?

J.D. Am I right in thinking that if you plot log flow rate against volume filtered, like I did, you get a straight line?

JF.S. Yes. I think they are the same results found by Gregersen *et al.* in 1966,

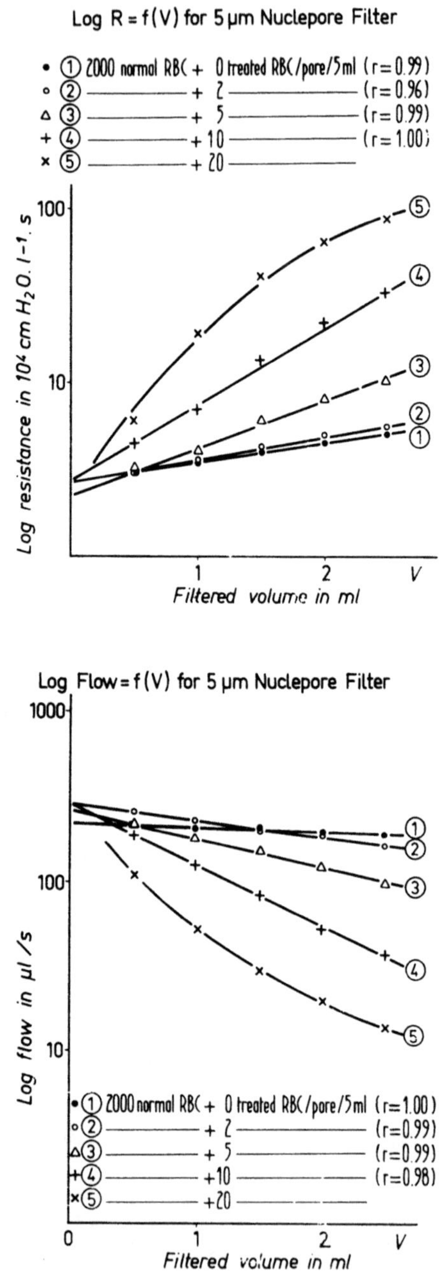

Log R = f(V) for 5 µm Nuclepore Filter
• ① 2000 normal RBC + 0 treated RBC/pore/5ml (r = 0.99)
∘ ② + 2 (r = 0.96)
Δ ③ + 5 (r = 0.99)
+ ④ + 10 (r = 1.00)
× ⑤ + 20
Log resistance in 10⁴ cm H₂O . l-1 . s
100
10
1
2
V
Filtered volume in ml
Log Flow = f(V) for 5 µm Nuclepore Filter
1000
100
10
Log flow in µl/s
• ① 2000 normal RBC + 0 treated RBC/pore/5ml (r = 1.00)
∘ ② + 2 (r = 0.99)
Δ ③ + 5 (r = 0.99)
+ ④ +10 (r = 0.98)
× ⑤ +20
0
1
2
V
Filtered volume in ml

Fig. 3.30

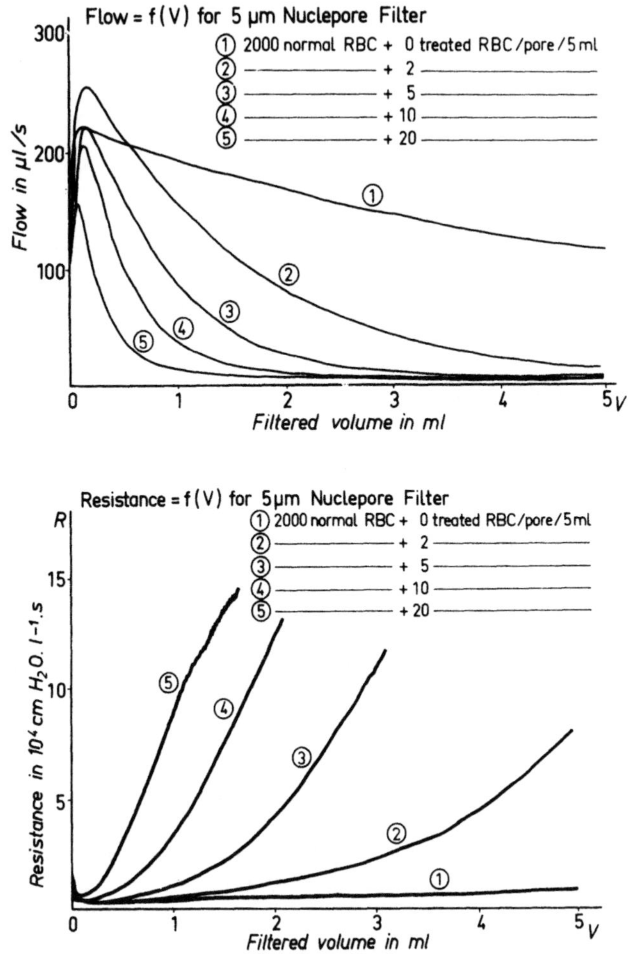

Fig. 3.31

but the haematocrit is very low because we used between 0.5 to 5 haematocrit.

P.G. John Stuart is next.

J.S. We have been trying to improve the positive-pressure filtration system I described this morning: that of Kenny *et al.* (1981) using 6 minutes' pumping time and measuring the filtration ratio of the pressure generated by washed red cells to the pressure generated by buffer alone. We remove the leucocytes by various pre-filtration techniques. Although you can remove 99% of the white cells fairly reliably, you certainly remove some of the reticulocytes and there is a risk of removing a subpopulation of stiff red cells as well. There may therefore be limitations to white cell removal techniques. We realised that there was another

Exponential regression (N = 10)				
$\frac{dV}{dt} = a_1 e^{b_1 V}$				
Number of treated RBC/pore/5 ml + 2000 normal RBC/pore/5 ml	2	5	10	20
R^2	0.99	0.99	0.98	0.90
a_1	285.9	282	300	158
b_1	−0.53	−1.04	−2.12	−2.54

Exponential regression (N = 10)				
Resistance $= a_2 e^{b_2 V}$				
Number of treated RBC/pore/5 ml + 2000 normal RBC/pore/5 ml	2	5	10	20
R^2	0.96	0.99	1.00	0.94
a_2	$2.66.10^4$	$2.23.10^4$	$2.73.10^4$	$4.3.10^4$
b_2	0.89	1.55	2.50	3.24

Fig. 3.32

way of compensating for the white cell count which I think is conceptually wrong, but I would like to show the method and the results we have obtained in one clinical situation.

The technique is to plot our red cell filtration ratio, that is the pressure above the filter during 6 minutes' pumping time, against the logarithm of the leucocyte count. The details are given in the paper that was circulated this afternoon (Stuart *et al.*, 1983, Filtration of washed erythrocytes in atherosclerosis and diabetes mellitus). What we did was to take 10 normal donors and do mixing experiments with their EDTA-anticoagulated blood, removing or adding buffy coat so that we achieved a range of leucocyte counts from 1.5–20.0 × 10^9/l for a total of 70 blood samples from the 10 donors. The red cell filtration ratio was then measured on each sample and this gave an overall correlation between the ratio and the logarithm of the leucocyte count for the 70 samples of $r = 0.653$ ($P < 0.001$). The regression line was then used to correct the red cell filtration ratio of individual patients for their own leucocyte count, just as one adjusts whole-blood viscosity for haematocrit.

This next slide (Fig. 3.33) shows the approach applied to a new study, which has been circulated this afternoon and is in press in *Clinical Hemorheology*, in which we took 55 steady-state male diabetic out-patients and compared them with 37 healthy controls matched for age and smoking. We found that the leucocyte count of our diabetics was 7% higher than that of the controls, although this was not statistically significant. If you look at the red cell filtration ratio, uncorrected for leucocyte count, then it is significantly higher in the diabetics compared with the controls, suggesting results similar to Dr Juhan's obtained in the uncontrolled diabetic; but I repeat that our patients were controlled diabetics in the out-patient clinic. When we adjusted for the leucocyte count to a standard count of 7.5×10^9/l, the difference disappeared and we think the leucocytosis was responsible for the initial result of a false high increase in red cell rigidity in diabetes. Some of these patients were then studied with a drug that has been claimed to increase intracellular cyclic AMP and thus increase red cell flexibility. The drug is ticlopidine and the next slide (Fig. 3.34) shows the results in 20 diabetics who were given placebo for 12 weeks and then ticlopidine for 12 weeks. We found that the uncorrected red cell filtration ratio at week 24 was significantly improved compared with week 12 but this 12 week treatment period was associated with a significant reduction in leucocyte count and in fact the drug has now been removed from the British market, at least temporarily, because it can cause neutropenia. So the message is that when you review a paper

	Diabetics (55)	p	Controls (37)
Leucocyte count ($\times 10^9$/l)	7.4±2.1	NS	6.9±1.6
Plasma viscosity (mPa s) at 25° C	1.66±0.12	NS	1.64±0.09
Whole blood viscosity (mPa s) at 25° C and 128 s^{-1}	6.24±0.46	NS	6.20±0.35
Red cell filtration (ratio)			
– uncorrected	4.03±0.79	<0.01	3.58±0.59
– adjusted for leucocyte count	4.29±1.53	NS	4.12±1.05

Fig. 3.33

	Week 1	Placebo p	Week 12	Ticlopidine p	Week 24
Leucocyte count ($\times 10^9$/l)	7.2±1.5	<0.05	7.8±1.8	<0.02	6.8±2.1
Red cell filtration (ratio)					
– uncorrected	3.95±0.69	NS	4.01±0.81	<0.05	3.42±0.70
– adjusted for leucocyte count	4.29±1.32	NS	3.71±1.23	NS	4.09±1.18

Fig. 3.34

claiming that a drug improves red cell deformability, please look hard at the effects of the drug on the leucocyte count.

The fundamental doubt, however, is that if you use regression lines for correction, unless your r value is 0.98 or 0.99, all your results are going to become artificially normal. With an r value of around 0.6, as in this case, obviously there is a lot of scatter on either side of that line, so you are using a very crude correction method. There may therefore be a real change in red cell deformability which this correction method masks.

H.M. I was lulled into a false sense of security which you have just shattered. Did you just say that you do not believe in your correction of leucocytes?

J.S. It obviously corrects for leucocytes, but I think it overcorrects. It is too crude a correction method.

H.M. To be more specific, the result of your leucocyte correction, for both the drug experiment and for the diabetics versus controls, was to eliminate any difference. Is that what you believe is the true case?

J.S. It certainly eliminated the obvious difference. There may yet be a true difference in erythrocyte deformability which our technique was not sensitive enough to detect. I think to do this properly you need a better r value – 0.65 is not good enough.

J.D. Your correction might actually hide a difference.

J.S. Yes that is right. We have corrected for a major variant, which is leucocyte count, but we may have hidden, as you say, a real change in red cell deformability.

G.L. Just to say, John, that you determine the area under the curve for up to 6 minutes, and it is therefore almost entirely determined by leucocyte plugging anyway. You cannot really say anything about that initial P_i, which is what we are interested in.

J.S. That is what you are interested in, yes. No I cannot say anything about it either.

P.G. Thank you very much and the next presentation will be by Dr Ehrly, please.

A.E. I am not a speciaist on platelets, but as a clinician one is impressed that patients who have trombocytosis with thrombocyte counts of 1 million have very low filtration rates, even when corrected to a haematocrit of 10%. There are other patients who have very low thrombocyte counts, and they have relatively high flow rates. It is, I think, generally accepted that platelets play a role in the filtration values independently of the method used. So I think it is very important to have a well-defined sampling technique as Dr Hanss has pointed out. I would like to describe what we did some year ago and what we are doing now in this respect. We take the fresh sample of blood, we take an aliquot of 1½ cc of blood without letting the buffy coat to be established, but we centrifugate the other part of the blood to obtain immediately about 13 cc of fresh plasma free of white cells and platelets. Then we mix the $1\frac{1}{2}$ cc of blood and the 13 cc of plasma. It is known that even during the settling process or if you make a centrifugation, the white cells and platelets will aggregate. If you have aggregates of white cells and platelets they will settle faster in the tube of blood. Using this technique we have found that it is sufficient to have this ratio between plasma and blood to eliminate the white cells and the platelets sufficiently so that the results of the measurements are not too bad.

P.G. Thank you very much. Anybody else who would like to comment on platelets? Did you use EDTA?

A.E. I have never tried experiments with EDTA. We use low dose heparin.

P.G. Then let us go on to a general discussion of these topics.

H.S-S. Is there anybody in this room who is willing to accept as an editor or as a private reader a paper in which whole blood is filtered and in which the text talks about red cell flexibility or some other similar term which relates to the rheology of red cells? Would this person please stand up and put this on record.

G.A.M. I have thought a lot about this problem and since about one year ago in the French Group we speak about blood microfiltration. I would suggest blood microfiltration, which is completely different from red cell deformability but nevertheless exists.

J.D. My answer to Holger's question is yes, if the author used the term red cell filtration. If he has a technique which gets a result within seconds, then I think it would be not unreasonable to talk about red cell filtration.

G.L. It depends on what context you are talking about, but if you have a journal called *Clinical Haemorheology* there is no doubt that blood microfiltration, or whatever you want to call it, has rheological aspects to it. If somebody comes up with a paper which has a clinical relevance, then I think that is quite reasonable. For example, I will present tomorrow briefly the Reid/Dormandy method and prediction of deep vein thrombosis. As it happens, it is of no value whatsoever but, just to give you a hypothesis, if it had showed a complete separation of patients who went on to get thrombosis and patients who did not, that would certainly have been interesting and the test has rheological aspects to it. And that kind of study, I think if it does show you something interesting, merits publication.

H.S-S. You would accept red cell deformability appearing in the text or in the caption?

G.L. I think I would ask the author to change the title of it.

P.G. If this finishes the general discussion, then Dr Chien is going to summarise.

S.C. This session deals with the effects of haematocrit, white cells and platelets on filterability. There is only one comment on platelets. Dr Ehrly showed that in patients with very high thrombocyte counts above 1 million, there is also a reduction in filterability. This is like the situation in the early days with white cells. The white cells were neglected for a long time and now they are being treated with equal rights with the red cells, maybe more so. Maybe one of these days we will do the same thing to the platelets.

As far as the red cells and the white cells are concerned, it is the general concensus that they have different filterability, the white cells being much more rigid than the red cells. When filtering a mixture of these cells, with time the effect of the white cells will become more and more dominant as they plug the pores, regardless of the technique that you use. Therefore, in order to get any information on the red cell deformability from filterability tests in the presence of white cells, the interpretation must be made with caution. Of course, the best solution is to remove as much of the white cells as possible, and several methods have been mentioned, e.g. repeated washing, the use of the Nakao filter, are some of the examples, but it is difficult to remove all the white cells, therefore, the interpretation becomes an important aspect.

Different filtration techniques have been used. Either you measure the pressure at a constant flow or you measure the flow at a constant pressure. Regardless of the method used, in order to determine red cell deformability one must use the early part of the curve, either the initial pressure reading at a constant flow or the initial flow at a constant pressure. Several techniques have been devised to obtain initial flow at a constant pressure. Dr Hanss has devised an instrument to get the very early reading on the flow at a constant pressure. Dr Dormandy has proposed to use two points later in the curve and extrapolate back to 0 time on a semilogarithmic curve. Dr Stoltz has devised a technique to continuously monitor the flow, and again you can get the 0 time flow behaviour at a constant pressure. Similarly, with the constant flow method one can read the initial pressure from the pressure time curve. Those pressure or flow readings then can be used to deduce a resistance factor, which is the pressure/flow ratio for the suspension. This should be normalised by the pressure/flow ratio for the suspending medium through the same filter to yield a relative resistance. Several investigators have calculated some intrinsic deformability of the red cells from such data by dividing the additional relative resistance of the suspension, which equals relative resistance minus 1, by the red cell concentration or the haematocrit. That is, the intrinsic viscosity type of concept is used to deduce an intrinsic parameter of red cell deformability. This parameter has been called an IF index or the Greek letter beta. This approach is a useful way to pull together all the data obtained by using different techniques.

We also have a problem of choosing what haematocrit to test. It seems that too high a haematocrit would cause the presence of more than one cell in a pore. Dr Dormandy's and our data both indicate that the haematocrit should be around 10% to 20%. If you go down too low, the problem is the possibility of an inaccuracy in measurement. If the measurement is accurate, you can go down even lower in haematocrit.

Now we turn to the white cells. In the later phase of the filtration curve, if white cells are present their influences are felt increasingly more with time. Therefore, the later phase is dominated by the white cells. Dr Skalak has proposed some theoretical ways to analyse, from the later phase of the curve, the influence of white cells on the filtration. From this one can get some idea of what percent of the white cells will plug up the filter and presumably one can also derive the white cell deformability from such tests. In a number of situations, including post-operative patients in pregnancy, diabetes and some drug treatments, Dr Buchan and Dr Stuart showed that there is a decrease in filterability and in some cases there is also pore plugging by white cells; the decrease in filterability in these various states may indeed be due to the white cell plugging. When one does long-term filterability tests, one has to be particularly aware of the probability that white cell plugging may dominate the picture. Among the white cells it appears that the granulocytes are more important in plugging than the other white cells. From these considerations the point has been made that whole blood filterability should not be made synonymous with red cell filterability. This is a summary of what the session on haematocrit, white cells and platelets do to the filtration test.

P.G. Thank you very much. We will immediately move on to the next session.

Plasma and suspending medium

P.G. The next part of this session deals with plasma factors and suspending medium and I will call on Dr Barnes to start.

A.B. Several years ago we carried out a pan investogram on a group of diabetic patients and a group of normal controls. Mean age of the 64 diabetics studied was 55; 61 control subjects had similar age, and sex distribution. They were about 15% over ideal body weight. One of the variables that we looked at was whole blood filtration by the Reid/Dormandy method, and I will show you a list of correlation coefficients for all the things that we measured against whole blood filtration. Of course, spurious correlations will come up one after another because of the large number of variables actually being measured. (Fig. 3.35) I have underlined the coefficients that come out as significant. In the diabetics there was no significance in glucose, electrolytes or protein concentrations in the plasma. Zinc, for some peculiar reason, and triglycerides come out as a positive, so the higher these levels the slower is the filtration; these correlations are, however, not significant in the normal group. There is a slight degree of correlation on total protein and albumin in the normals. There is no correlation in the viscosity

Correlation coefficients for filtration and chemical and rheological variables

	Diabetics	Normals		Diabetics	Normals
Glucose	0.135	0.032	Cholesterol	0.053	0.048
Urea	0.072	0.077	Triglycerides	<u>0.301</u>	0.015
Creatinine	0.052	0.130	Phospholipid	0.062	0.156
Protein total	0.053	<u>0.318</u>	ESR	0.187	0.048
Albumin	0.063	<u>0.312</u>	PCV	0.104	<u>0.265</u>
Globulin	0.130	0.185	MDA	0.149	0.246
Caeruloplasmin	0.222	0.034	Visc 0.77	0.118	0.029
Fibrinogen	0.135	0.207	Visc 2.62	0.023	<u>0.277</u>
Cu	0.170	0.014	Visc 23	0.013	0.126
Zn	<u>0.296</u>	0.082	Visc 230	0.062	0.118

Fig. 3.35

results. This slide (Fig. 3.36) shows the correlation between filtration and clinical variables. There is a significant correlation with body weight in the normals but not in the diabetics; so that the heavier the normals are, the slower their blood filters. Rather surprisingly the correlation with blood pressure came out quite well, so that you can actually estimate blood pressure by filtering whole blood. Thank you very much.

P.G. Questions or comments to this presentation? Thank you very much Adrian. The next speaker is Dr Hanss.

M.H. In our search to have the best experimental conditions for filtration measurements we have done experiments to show the influence of some variables on the results. This slide (Fig. 3.37) plots the relative variation of the filtration index, ($\triangle$IF) versus pH, using the value at pH 7.4 as the normal value for comparison. There is an increase of the cell rigidity both on the basic and the acidic side. We do not know why. However, we just want to say that you can allow for fluctuations of a few tenths of pH units around physiological level without affecting the filtration. I have shown this morning the temperature effects, which on the contrary are rather critical. Another factor which we have studied is the osmolality, which was changed by varying the sodium chloride content. The normal physiological level is taken to be 300 mOsm. The filtration index rises very steeply on either side of the physiological level (Fig. 3.38). So it is more important to control the osmolality than pH in the suspending medium. The small spots are viscosity measurements inside the red blood cells, and I am a bit surprised by the figure Shu Chien told us about what was the figure you gave? (*S.C.*: 7 centipoises). We got about 3 centipoises measured by electron spin resonance inside the red blood cell. We have not done the experiment, we have used other people's determinations. The sphericity index calculated from cell surface area and volume is also shown to explain the osmolality effects. Then we tried to determine the influence of oxygen and carbon dioxide contents. On normal blood samples the IF figures are independent of the oxygen content of the suspending medium. Of course, when you have abnormal haemoglobin it is not the same. It is not necessary to control the oxygen content unless you suspect haemoglobin disorders. The red blood cell becomes slightly more rigid when the

Correlation coefficients for filtration and clinical variables

	Diabetics	Normals		Diabetics	Normals
Age	0.157	0.014	Syst BP	0.069	0.389
Weight	0.107	0.373	Dias BP	0.243	0.479
Duration	0.127	0.000	Cap frag L	0.064	0.090
Smoking	0.061	0.403	Cap frag R	0.077	0.297

Fig. 3.36

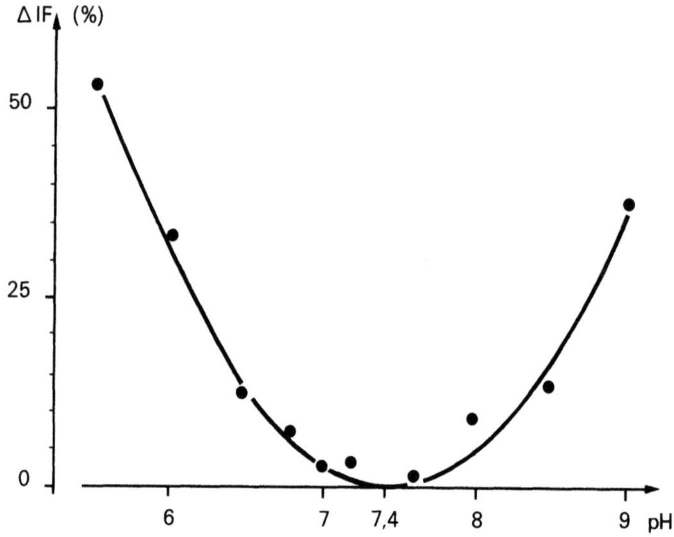

Fig. 3.37

CO_2 content increases above the physiological level, which may be important in some physiological or physio-pathological conditions. Thank you.

P.G. Questions.

H.M. A question about the osmolality. The data look very symmetric around the isotonic region. Yet there are other publications indicating that red cells are much more sensitive to swelling than they are to shrinking. Can you comment on that?

M.H. Yes. We did not use the same filtration index which has been used in other experiments. Our index is directly proportional to the red blood cell property. I think this may be the difference.

S.F. Using whole blood we observed the same behaviour you had for osmolality and for pH: symmetric in alkalosis and acidosis and in hypotonic and hypertonic solutions.

P.T. I would like to make a very short comment about the symmetry of these changes around the iso-osmality. According to our experience it is extremely variable according to the diameter of the pore which is utilised. Symmetries are found when working with 3 micron pores, which are more sensitive to swelling and not to shrinking. For larger pores the opposite is true, i.e. then the greater sensitivity is toward modification of internal viscosity; when red cells are swollen they flow better and they flow worse when they are shrunk by hypertonicity. Therefore the influence of the surface area to volume relationship on so-called red cell deformability has to be related to the geometry of the system in which this

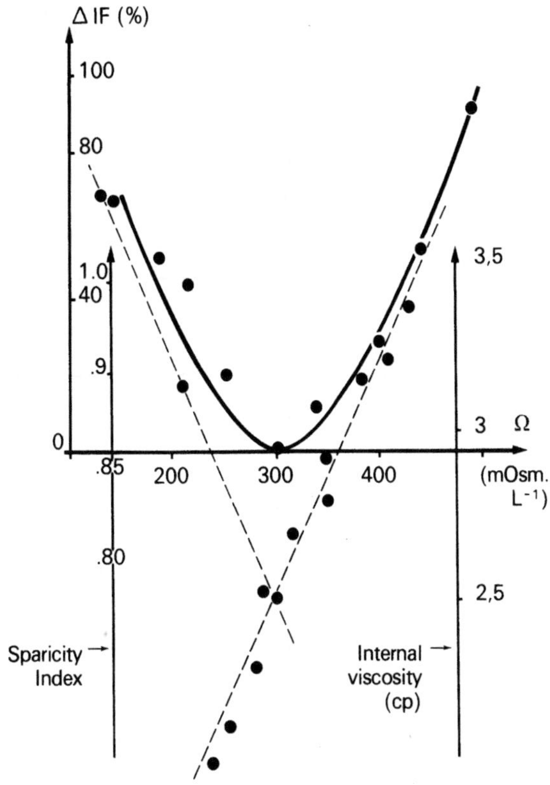

Fig. 3.38

test is being performed.

S.C. We have obtained data on red cell filterability versus pH essentially the same as that shown by Dr Hanss. Any change in deformability could be due to changes in membrane, changes in the internal viscosity or the shape. I think with pH you do have some shape change when you go to extreme pH values. We also measured the internal fluid viscosity, the haemoglobin viscosity, and found it to be not much affected by pH over the range of our experiments. But the membrane viscosity of the red cell changes as determined by using a micropipette varies similarly to the whole cell filterability. Usually we think that the internal fluid viscosity is more dominant in this filterability test, but in this case it appears that the membrane change is correlated with the whole cell filterability.

M.H. I believe membrane properties are dominant in the normal red blood cell deformability. (*S.C.*: In this case they certainly correlate.) Yes, but we have many experiments with ghosts and had the same filtration rate as for the whole cell.

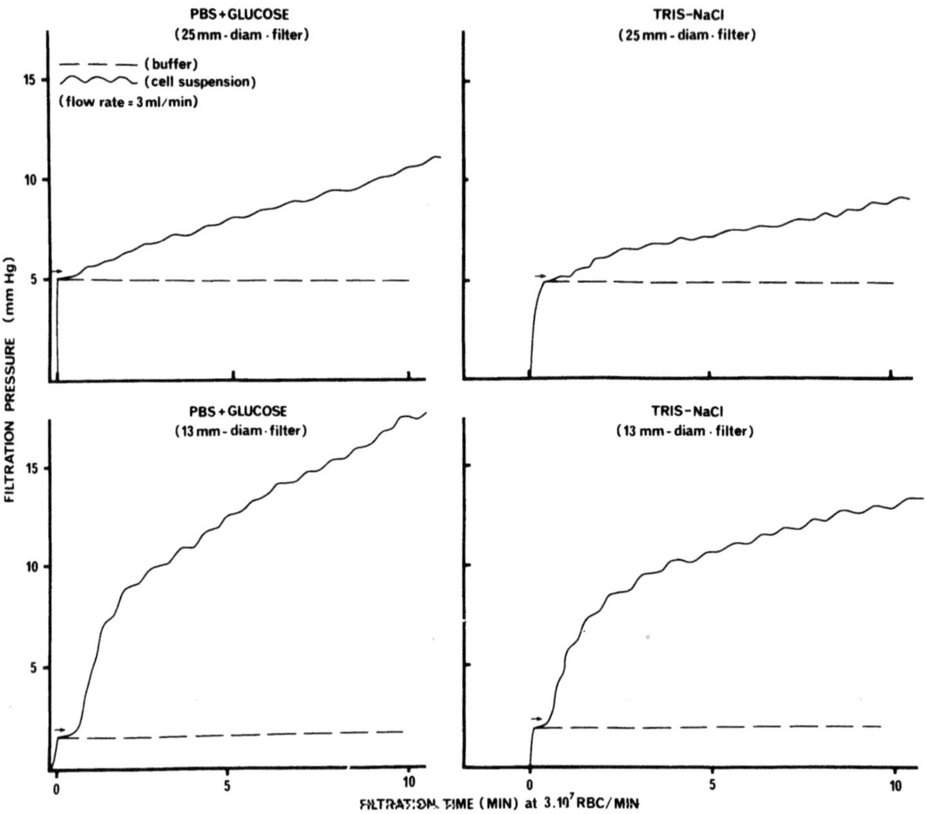

Fig. 3.39

P.G. Thank you very much. We now move on to Pierre Leblond's presentation.

P.L. Just two points I want to illustrate with this slide (Fig. 3.39) showing four actual tracings of filtration pressure at a constant flow. Cells were washed and suspended in two kinds of buffer for filtration. The curves on the left were done with phosphate buffered saline: pH 7.4, 300 mOsm plus 5% glucose. The curves on the right were obtained with tris sodium chloride 10 mmol tris. The upper tracings were obtained with use of the 25 mm diameter Nuclepore membranes with a 3 micron pore diameter and a low pore density, those are the ones we call our special membranes which we cannot obtain anymore. We thought it might be good to try to work also with standard membranes, and so we purchased the smaller 13 mm membranes with the standard pore density for 3 micron diameter pores. The first phenomenon I would like to show you is what I was relating to this morning. The flow rate in the system is the same for all tracings. The flat tracings represent base line resistance obtained for buffer. We expected that the resistance ratio of cells to buffer would be about the same for the large and small membranes. It turned out to be quite different. The small membranes have low resistance for buffer but they have a high resistance ratio of cells to buffer as compared to the larger membranes with a lower pore density. I think it has to do with this entrance phenomenon or geometrical conditions as the cells enter the pore. The other point I would like to make, which is more pertinent to this session, that the cell resistance is lower in phosphate glucose than in tris, and this was much more pronounced with the small 13 mm membranes. If we calculate the cell/buffer resistance index, either at the end of filtration or from the initial values, it is almost a factor of 40% difference between the two types of buffer. So we decided on that basis to continue filtering in phosphate plus glucose. My only interpretation at this moment is that using tris sodium chloride, by the time you have washed the cells and shovelled them around the lab until they get to filtration you may have altered their deformability on the basis of some metabolic breakdown somewhere; whereas maybe with the phosphate buffer with glucose added you protect them somewhat better.

S.C. Pierre, is the difference due to the glucose or due to the phosphate versus tris?

P.L. We have tried phosphate alone. We did get part of this change but it seems that when we add glucose we have even better, so we moved a step further and included glucose all alone.

P.G. Thank you very much. We then proceed to the last presentation by Holger Schmid-Schonbein.

H.S-S. I would like to start with what I said at the last meeting when I reported the evolution of our filtration test. Slide (Fig. 3.40). We were using one of the commercially available filter holders, the Milipore filter holder, and put in 25 mm diameter Nuclepore sieves. We were interested in coming down to low driving pressures for obvious reasons. We suspended 10% red cells in plasma and found an extremely poor reproducibility. We could have 0 flow very often. And then we looked at the pores and of course we saw the bouquet formation, at the lower end of the sieve, but we also had some at the upper end. In other words, we saw clogging of red cell aggregates, trying to enter two or three at a time into the pores. So we redesigned the system and (slide) (Fig. 3.41) we had at the end of this little funnel a recess to create a lateral flow, and with that immediately we coped with that problem. And we come up with a figure for the relative flow rate of the suspension (10% haematocrit) divided by the flow rate of the suspending medium of roughly 0.7. If we calculate the IF from that, we are off by a factor of 3 from the same parameter in Dr Hanss' system using the old traditional approach of having the red cells sort of falling into each of the pores. We think this is a very important thing one has to study more. We had Dr Hanss' system, but unfortunately we had to give it back, but we plan to redesign this system using this. This is important because obviously there is a place for leaving the red cells in

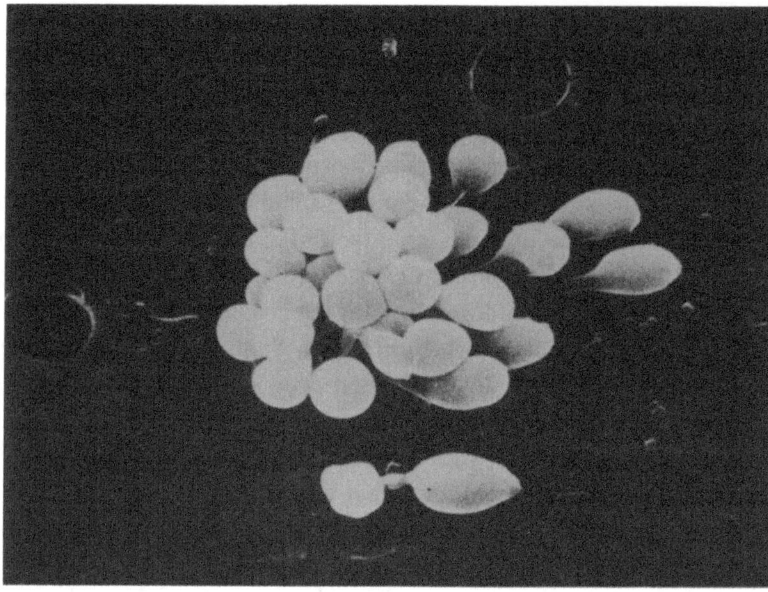

Fig. 3.40

3. Step:

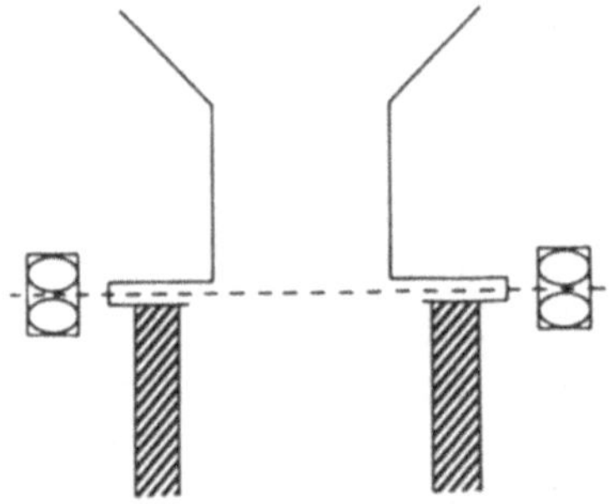

Attempt to improve flow conditions for RBC entry into pores

$\dot{V}_{rel}$ of 10 % RBC in plasma		(S.D./$\bar{x}$)
150 mm H_2O	0.690 ± 0.08	0.178
50 mm H_2O	0.685 ± 0.059	0.171

Fig. 3.41

their plasma, irrespective of the question of the anticoagulant. We were looking at the red cells in plasma, and of course we find especially in patients an extreme tendency to aggregation and therefore also very rapid sedimentation. We know from our own results as well as those from Harry Goldsmith that as you reduce the haematocrit the forces needed to disperse red cell aggregates, the classical rouleau formation, go up very high. We still do not have a good technique even to measure that at the moment, either by viscometry or photometry. We have shown in diabetics that very small micro-aggregates form at very high shear rates and they are difficult to disperse. They sediment in lower shear conditions and resist high shear stresses and I will show you that in a minute, that these affect the filtration measurement as soon as we have a low pressure and a low shear on the cells as they enter. Therefore the chance of cell triplets, quadruplicates, etc., trying to enter the pore at once is a very substantial one, which has not been talked about. And this of course is all related to plasma proteins. We know for example that this type of aggregation (clumps) is primarily formed by the presence of alpha 2 macroglobulin, whereas another type of aggregate (rouleaux) is formed primarily by fibrinogen. Using 8 micron Millipore filters in the old Millipore system, we did a large study with Roe Wells, which we published at the Heidelberg meeting of Congress of Haemorheology, that the ability of cells to pass through them was not affected by myocardial infarction. My system was used by various clinicians and most of all by E. Volger (slide) (Fig. 3.42), who found that in myocardial infarction there is a certain difference, but no more than maybe a 10% decrease. He also looked into the time course, and his results are in striking discrepancy to some of the data that have been published elsewhere. (Slide) (Fig. 3.43) We therefore again took our SER, and in this slide 1 is unwashed cells in buffer, 2 is washed cells, 3 is the cells in their serum, 4 the cells in their plasma. The cells in the suspending medium with a lower viscosity would tend to have a lower mean passage time, so we corrected these for the continuous phase viscosity. You now see that, with the exception of the washed cells, the normal cells in saline, the cells in plasma or the cells in serum have about the same mean passage time; in other words we have no evidence from this type of study that the plasma proteins affect the deformability directly, and this is in keeping with what I said this morning. This is borne out even more in the next experiment in which we used fibrinogen of various concentrations, covering the whole range which is clinically interesting. We found that in the buffer without correction we have about 20% lower passage time; now if this passage time is corrected for the viscosity of the medium, there is no indication of any type of a red cell rigidification over this very dramatic increase in fibrinogen concentration. So with this background and especially in the light of the controversy about the abnormalities in Raynaud's disease patients, where we feel very strongly that the cells are normal in most cases but strongly aggregated and John Dormandy has voiced the opposite, we felt that we should look at this in

	Control group	Coronary heart disease	p
Aggregation of erythrocytes			
Resistance to splitting	2.45±0.49	3.38±0.76	<0.005
τ_{Tmin} (dyn · cm^{-2})			
n	40	50	
Corrected size of aggregation in stasis,	0.25±0.06	0.73±0.25	<0.005
$\lambda \cdot \eta_{pl}$ (dyn · cm^{-2} · 10^{-2})			
n	54	50	
Relation of aggregation in prestasis and stasis, FSAR	0.89±0.02	0.88±0.03	n.s.
n	55	50	
Deformability of erythrocytes			
relative filtration rate	0.63±0.08	0.59±0.07	<0.05
$\dot{V}_{rel}$			
n	21	19	

From Volger 1980

Fig. 3.42

more detail. We should really look into the effect of red cell aggregation in the filtration tests which are now in use, in which we have only low shear stresses, therefore the chance of red cell aggregate dispersion is of course becoming small. So we did a very simple experiment (slide) (Fig. 3.44). I still had an old Brookfield and we took a large Millipore sieve and designed a little system in which I can now filter cell suspension while they are being sheared. The rest of the apparatus is a very small flow meter. The studies were done with various driving pressures which were essentially the difference between the fluid level and the exit. Of course, we have some corrections to be made for some interfacial effects, but they will not change the dramatic difference which we see on the next slide (Fig. 3.45). The samples are 10% red cells in our buffer, which contains 0.25% albumin, and the cells of the same donor heparinised in his own plasma. This is a log scale and you can see that as we have aggregation whether we shear, expecially if we do not shear, we have this dramatic fall in the flow rates from an initial fairly high level to very low levels. The majority of samples come to a stop. We can always avoid the stop if we shear the sample above it. We have none of these problems if we use these same cells in buffer. The interesting thing is the flow rates go down, but they go down very very slowly. This is in the midst of a study, but what you see is that if one has red cells in buffer and shears, you can completely avoid plugging. If

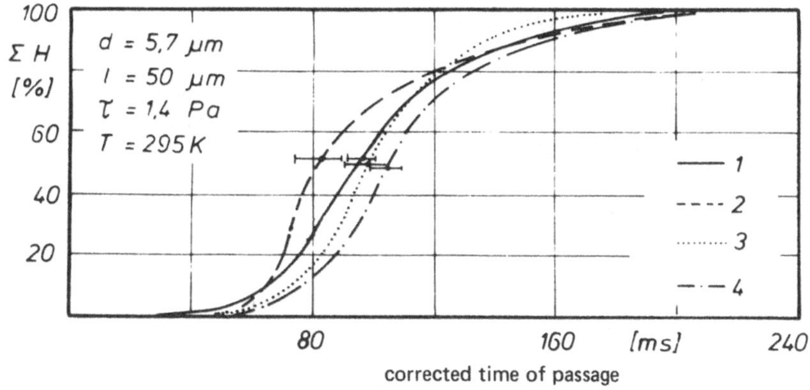

Fig. 3.43

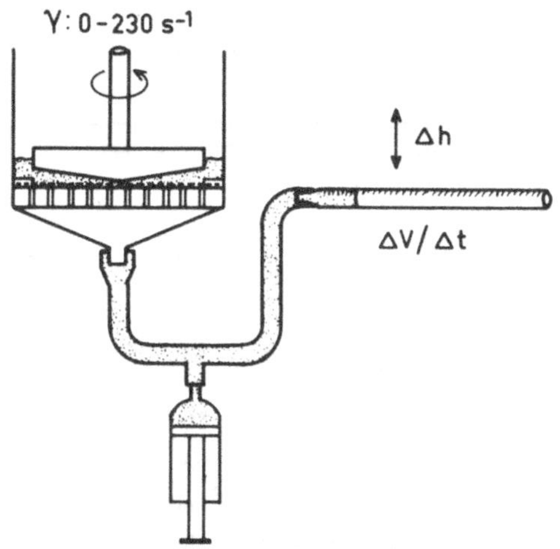

Fig. 3.44

anything, the flow rate goes up higher. So we are talking about an entrance effect here which is strongly related to the plasma, and we believe the plasma proteins causing red cell aggregation. If it is a 3 minute experiment you can see that the absence of shearing, i.e. the absence of hydrodynamic forces that disperse at least in part these red cell aggregates, these precipitous drops in the flow rate would seem to be clogging. But we are not quite sure it is clogging alone. It could also be that we are beginning to see a scum of cells which rest above the filter. In any event, these data indicate that the absolute values here are 10 to 20 times higher

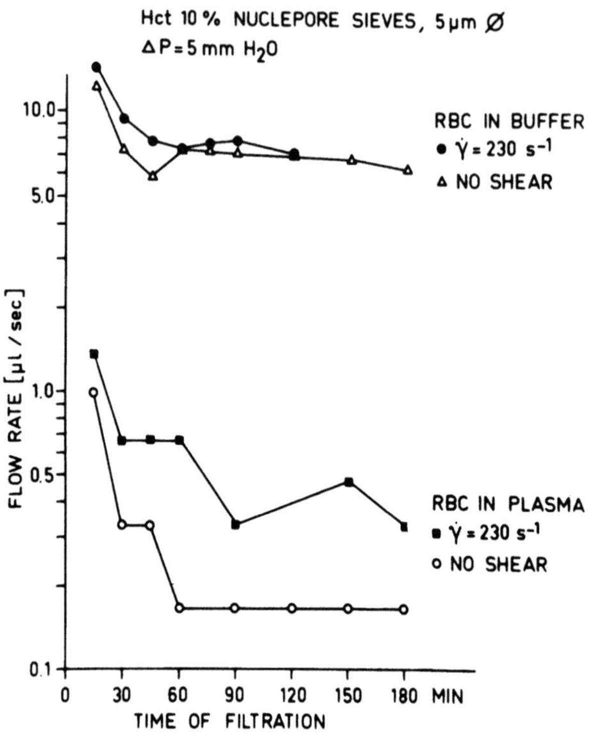

Fig. 3.45

and that these effects are in fact of major significance in the evaluation of filtration experiments with low pressure. Thank you very much.

M.H. In the last slide, were they constant shear stress or constant shear rates?

H.S-S. Constant shear stress. Constant pressure, as good as we could.

M.H. Were they rotated at the same speed?

H.S-S. Yes, always 230 sec^{-1}.

M.H. So it is not constant shear stress.

H.S-S. We now have to differentiate between the shear stress in the sample and the shear stress at the pore.

M.H. In the sample.

H.S-S. In the sample it was always 230 reciprocal seconds, that is roughly 0.2 or 0.3 pascals, and the 5 mm water gives you 50 pascals at the pore entrance.

P.G. I will turn the meeting over to Dr Chien to summarise this part.

S.C. This session is entitled plasma factors and suspending medium. Part of it was already dealt with this morning in relation to anticoagulants. We have discussed the effects of changing the suspending medium on the filterability. As far as pH is concerned, there seems to be an optimum at 7.4. The optimum osmolality is 300 mOsm. Both of these are physiological conditions. If we change the pH or osmolality in either direction there will be a reduction in the filterability of the sample. It was pointed out that the dependence of filterability on osmolality is a function of the geometry of the channel, i.e. filters with different pore sizes may have different optima. Variations in oxygenation of the sample do not have any influence on filterability of normal red cells, a high CO_2 level may reduce filterability. The phosphate buffered saline plus glucose provides a better filterability than tris saline; this is probably due in part to the phosphate buffer itself and in part to the glucose. The presence of macromolecules such as fibrinogen in the suspending medium can increase red cell aggregation, and this may reduce the filterability. Comparison of the filterability of a sample in plasma under shear to that without shear has shown that the shear dispersion of the aggregates helps to maintain the filterability at a better level than without shear. In buffer, where there is no red cell aggregation, the shearing of the suspension before the filtration does not make such a significant difference. In normal subjects and diabetic patients correlations of various plasma factors and clinical variables with whole blood filterability show that not many parameters are

Order of the influence of various factors on filtration methods

Method/Order	Method I	Method II	Method III	Method IV	Method V
Intrinsic flow property of red cell	7	3	1	1	1
Property of red cell secondary to plasma factor	4	1	7	7	2
Variability of filter	2	5	4	4	5
White cell or platelet effect	1	2	2	2	3
Storage effect	3	4	3	3	4
Effect of temperature or pH	6	7	5	5	7
Anticoagulant effect	5	6	6	6	6

Filtration methods

Method I	Whole blood. Positive water pressure. Measure of flow rate
Method II	Red cells in plasma. Atmospheric pressure. Haematocrit $<20\%$. Compared to plasma alone
Method III	Red cells in buffer. Constant pressure. Haematocrit $<20\%$. Compared to buffer alone
Method IV	Red cells in buffer. Constant flow rate. Haematocrit $<20\%$. Compared to buffer alone
Method V	Red cells in plasma. Constant flow rate. Haematocrit $<20\%$. Compared to plasma alone

Fig. 3.46

significantly correlated. In diabetic patients the triglyceride and zinc levels and diastolic blood pressure were correlated with filterability; in the controls total protein concentration, haematocrit, weight, smoking and blood pressure were correlated with whole blood filterability. It is surprising that fibrinogen and haematocrit did not show better correlation. In summary, in order to get reproducible filterability tests the suspending medium must be controlled with respect to pH, osmolality, and the degree of red cell aggregation, in order to avoid the complicating effects of the variations in these factors on filterability.

P.G. Thank you very much Dr Chien. I think that very nicely sums up what we have heard this afternoon. I would like just to mention the questionnaire which has been passed around and which is an anonymous poll that Dr Marcel and Dr Dormandy would like you to complete. You are here asked to indicate the importance of various factors contributing to the result of a filtration measurement. You all probably remember Tony Marcel's cake diagram, where he had indicated in a circle the various factors that to a varying degree affect the result of such a measurement and he has under the influence of various psychologists modified this drawing from a cake type to a stick or railway type of system and you are kindly asked to fill this out also.

(Thirteen forms were completed in full and Fig. 3.46 analyses the replies in terms of the significance of various factors and the results obtained by using five different methods of filtration. So, for instance, using whole blood filtration under positive pressure the consensus was that the most important influence on the result was the white cell or platelet effect and that the intrinsic property of the red cell was the least important).

SESSION 4

Types of filters

P.G. The first topic on our list for today is a discussion of types of filters. To begin with, Dr Schmid-Schönbein will show his film on RBC behaviour *in vitro* and *in vivo*.

H.S.-S. I was pleased to see that Dr Richard Skalak wants to measure how a red cell passes or glides through a 5 μ pore, in other words how the red cell adapts itself to the specific flow conditions that prevail when it approaches, enters and passes such a pore.

We know that mammalian red cells are unique in being able to adapt themselves to the flow of the continuous phase in which they are suspended, because their membrane can, as we say 'tank tread', i.e. transmit shear stresses into their cytoplasm.

I would like to point out to another very important factor contributing to RBC 'flexibility', namely to the viscosity of the membrane. We now have very strong evidence that in RBC containing unstable haemoglobins (the suspensions of which are notoriously stiff and poorly filterable) and also in RBC of diabetics under poor metabolic control, there is a considerable interaction between haemoglobin and spectrin. We have every reason to assume that in these cells the membrane viscosity will be abnormally high.

In analyzing what is going on with a cell as it passes through a pore in the filter, it is important to consider *the way it moves*: there are of course different possible mechanisms by which the gliding of the cells into and then through a pore in a Nuclepore sieve can be interfered with. Just assume that there is an additional cell hanging to the first one at the pore entrance (i.e. a two cell aggregate); then of course the tank treading of each membrane becomes extremely difficult if not impossible. If we have red cell aggregation (which is typical in many diseases associated with poor red cell filterability), then the entry of one individual RBC into a pore is likely to be disturbed.

Now the tank treading motion of the membrane can be analyzed in various ways. We have done it in viscometric flow (with the rheoscope) and together with Dr Peter Gaehtgens also in tube flow (with a moving glass capillary system).

This motion can also be analyzed in different other rheological setups, and we feel that these should also be utilized in parallel to filtration experiments. If, for example, you simply take red cells and pack them to anything above 60%, you will find that highly concentrated RBC suspensions have a remarkable low viscosity. This can only be explained by accepting the idea that there must be tank treading in flowing packed cells, a process which Dr Tim Secomb and Dr Richard Skalak are now analyzing theoretically. If we begin to appreciate that the tank treading of the membrane is important for the normal flow behaviour of RBC, we will also have to consider more carefully what types of filter we are using. In this context I would like to stress that indeed it is not sufficient to have only a good, i.e. well-defined *geometrical* model of a short capillary. Hydrodynamically, Nuclepore sieves are bad models of the microcirculation.

Let me remind you of the main conclusions of the comparative methodological study we presented here last year. The only good correlation we have been able to find in this study was between Nuclepore 'filterability' and the number of red cells which refused to enter into the single pore of the '*S*ingle *E*rythrocyte *R*igidometer' (SER) (so-called 'occluding cells'). This finding strongly suggested that individual pore occlusion is the main determinant of Nuclepore 'filterability'.

Now we feel that the tank treading mechanism is also essential for the normal behaviour of red cells *in vivo* and I am going to show you some new strips of film to document it.

This scene has been taken quasi *in vivo* with 200 frames per second in an isolated mesentery perfused with red cell suspensions. The erythrocytes are always asymmetrically deformed as they move at high shear rates along the straight main capillary. In addition, you can also observe the very particular behaviour of red cells as they arrive at the level of a so-called 'flow divider' at the branching point of a secondary capillary. This behaviour strongly suggests that membrane tank treading of adjacent cells might be involved in the mechanisms determining the entry of an individual cell into the branched capillary. Apparently only tank treading cells are actually diverted into the secondary vessel. Aspects seen in this last scene make us now feel that it would also be necessary to have a theoretical analysis of the RBC motion at the level of a flow divider.

To conclude: as we are trying to predict from *in vitro* measurements the behaviour of red cells in the living microcirculation, we will also have to understand this behaviour in more complex situations. We do not necessarily have to restrict ourselves to a simple geometric model of one unbranched capillary, but will probably also have to consider more complex models, closer to the geometric flow conditions likely to be encountered by red cells *in vivo*.

This is all I wanted to show you here.

P.G. Thank you very much. Anyone wish to comment or ask a question?

J.S. Two questions. How were the Heinz bodies produced in these cells? Did the experimental manipulation not cause erythrocyte membrane damage as well?

H.S-S. Heinz bodies have been produced in normal red cells by incubating them with acetyl-phenylhydrazine. Following this treatment the cells are really damaged, but there is no other way to demonstrate the phenomenon. The Heinz bodies were either freely floating inside the cytoplasm, or bound to the internal membrane face; so there is also a certain extent of membrane damage. We have also demonstrated the membrane tank treading with latex particles attached to the outer side of the membrane, and the motion is very similar.

J.S. Presumably it would be easy to get one patient with congenital Heinz body anaemia, or somebody post-splenectomy to do the same study on tank treading, just for confirmation. The other thing I wanted to ask is why do you postulate in diabetes that there is an interaction between haemoglobin and spectrin? You have glycosylation of both haemoglobin and membrane proteins and the two things have the same common cause but are independent.

H.S-S. That is absolutely true. I am just quoting recent additional evidence obtained by Tillmann and showing that in poorly controlled diabetes there is haemoglobin attached to the RBC membranes; this can be seen macroscopically and also on SDS gel electrophoresis of isolated membrane proteins. At the cytoplasmic side of the RBC membrane we have two extremely concentrated protein systems, namely spectrin and haemoglobin, which under normal conditions do not interact with one another. Dr Michael Sheetz has postulated that the normal phosphorylation of both haemoglobin and spectrin is the essential condition in preventing this abnormal interaction.

P.G. Thank you very much. I think we should now move on and Dr Paul Teitel will be the next speaker.

P.T. I considered that the presentation of the film Dr Schmid-Schönbein has just shown us would be appropriate in the context of the discussion to follow. It documented the tank treading motion of the membrane of flowing RBC, which *is not necessarily associated with an actual shape change*, i.e. actual 'deformation' (Scand. J. Clin. Lab. Invest., 1981, Suppl. 156 to vol. *141*; 13). In addition it showed the RBC behaviour, i.e. flow pattern, motion, deformation and interaction with the vessel wall at the level of a capillary branching *in vivo*, a behaviour which probably is one out of several important mechanisms ensuring a *homogenous* RBC distribution in the microcirculation. It is my feeling that this very point has not yet received the attention it deserves.

During preparation of this session on 'Types and Characteristics of Filters', I encountered some difficulties in obtaining contributions. Utilisation of polycarbonate Nuclepore® filters to assess RBC 'deformability' – regarded as an intrinsic physical cell 'property' – is currently so widespread, that a discussion of other types of filters could appear somehow obsolete at a first approach. Since, however, we developed in Aachen an automatic microcomputer-assisted measuring instrument in which now *any kind* of filter can be utilized, we thought it worthwhile to take a closer look at differences existing between various filters.

Based on the feeling that different filters and methods do not necessarily illuminate the same rheological features of the flowing RBC, we considered that such a discussion could contribute to a better understanding of what we are trying to measure.

A. Geometric and fluid dynamic conditions in different filtration setups

Generally speaking any modern rheological instrumentation comprises two main components: a flow chamber and peripheral equipment. The latter is designed to pick up measurement data and process them in different (more or less elaborate) ways. In recent years great progress has been achieved in developing peripheral equipment, but unfortunately not in developing the actual flow chamber.

In any type of flow chamber two main sets of parameters have to be well defined: geometric conditions and fluid dynamic conditions. The geometric conditions bear not only on the flow chamber proper (in terms of shape and dimensions) but also on its mounting and the configuration of the inflow and outflow conduits.* The dynamic conditions are: pressure differential between inflow and outflow levels of the flow chamber, shear stress and shear rate produced in the flow chamber (and the spatial distribution of their substantive values), linear flow velocity inside the flow chamber (and velocity profile), and important for particulate bodies in suspension, the duration of shear inside the flow chamber.

These two sets of conditions will concurrently determine (1) the *flow pattern*, i.e. streamline profile and trajectories of suspended particles, and (2) the motions and type of shape changes of these particles. Flow pattern and particle motions have to be defined not only for the actual passage through the flow chamber proper, but also for the region of approach and entry into, as well for the region of exit from the flow chamber,

In addition, the fluid analysed should be defined with respect to its structure and/or homogeneity, i.e. volume concentration of particulate bodies (haematocrit) and absence or presence (including concentration) of aggregating macromolecules in the continuous phase.

Filtration setups described in the literature differ to a great extent from one another with respect to these parameters. One should be aware of this and when reporting data always specify the conditions of measurement.

In filtration setups, the flow chamber consists essentially of one microscopi-

* These important data should not be neglected (as they frequently are), since they determine decisive phenomena in regions of transition.

cal narrow tube (MNT) in the filter membrane.* Polycarbonate Nuclepore® microsieves are considered to contain geometrically very well-defined MNT. Glass capillary arrays (Galileo Electro-Optics Corp., Sturbridge, Mass., U.S.A.) and VECO micro-precision sieves produced by electroforming and photo-etching (Veco Zeefplatenfabriek N.V., Eerbeek, Holland) have also well defined and in addition uniformly arrayed MNT. Other types of filters utilized for RBC filtration have channels with poor geometric definition. These include: paper filters i.e. meshworks of cellulose fibers (Schleicher & Schull GmbH, D-3354, Dassel, West Germany), Millipore filters (Millipore Filter Corportion, Bedford, Mass., U.S.A.) and metal membranes made of sintered silver granules (Selas Flotronics, Spring House, Pa., U.S.A.). With these filters it is more appropriate to speak of 'equivalent microscopic tubes' (EMT) instead of actual pores: approximate values for density, length and diameter of the EMT can be derived by calibrating these filters with Newtonian fluids of known density.

With any kind of filter membrane the most important fluid dynamic condition is the pressure differential driving the fluid through one microscopical narrow tube. Unfortunately, more often than not, this fact is disregarded, although it seems that in recent years an increasing number of investigators are becoming aware of it.

Let us now consider the wall shear stresses. In a microscopical narrow tube of 5 microns in diameter and 12 microns in length, the pressure head of 20 cm water column will produce a wall shear stress approximating 2000 dynes/cm^2 (200 Pa); in the single pore of the 'single erythrocyte rigidometer' the wall shear stress amounts to approximately 30 dynes/cm^2 (3 Pa) and in one EMT in the polymicroviscometric (PMV) approach with paper filters its starting value is approx. 20 dynes/cm^2 (2 Pa) and goes down to zero. As can be seen, the differences are of two orders of magnitude, and this is indeed considerable.

Which range of shear stresses should then be reasonably chosen for relevant measurements? We will all agree that a shear stress of 2000 dynes/cm^2 is well beyond the maximal value occurring physiologically in the circulation. We have also to be aware of the reports available in the literature showing that such high shear stresses do inflict some damage to red cells and eventually haemolyse them, even if the exposure times are relatively short. Consequently, measurements of the filter resistance increments at constant flow rates over several minutes – during which the wall shear stresses in the non-clogged MNT can easily exceed this value – should be evaluated with extreme caution with respect to their microcirculatory relevance. If we accept on the other hand the basic notion that rheological factors are becoming pathyphysiologically pivotal only in a disturbed microcirculation associated with a low flow state, it will stand to reason that

* To avoid confusion, utilization of the term 'capillary' should be restricted for the smallest blood vessels of the microcirculation.

relevant information will be obtained at shear stresses smaller than the minimal normal values. Realistically, we have also to appreciate the fact that red cells present a non-Newtonian flow behaviour even in the absence of aggregation. In other words, that *real* and small changes in their normal ability to deform and/or flow will be obvious in the first place at small values of shear stresses and will tend to disappear at high ones. What we are actually looking for is a *pathologic potential* which becomes operational only in low flow conditions, while irrelevant in normal ones.

The real problem we have to deal with is to understand what happens to red cells as they go through a flow chamber represented by one microscopical narrow tube and to appreciate to what extent these phenomena also take place in the living microcirculation. We would have to analyse the behaviour of a red cell while being in the following different flow situations 'extra vivum': approaching the entry of a MNT, entering it, actually passing through it and finally leaving it. Description of the motion of one RBC in these different steps of 'filter passage' is closely linked to problems of terminology. What do we actually have to measure when assessing what is still loosely termed RBC 'deformability'? Resistance of the membrane to bending, to shearing or the extension, its ability to tank tread, time-dependent relaxation phenomena, the viscosity of the cytoplasm, or globally the extent to which a RBC can adapt to the forces of flow? (Schmid-Schönbein & Gaehtgens, Scand. J. Clin. Lab. Invest., *41*, Suppl. 156: 13, 1981). In this respect our understanding of RBC 'filtrability' through Nuclepore microsieves is still incomplete.

Typical stereoscan electron micrographs of one single RBC entering into a 'pore' of a Nuclepore filter (such as Fig. 9 in: Schröer R. & Muth K., La Ricerca Clin. Lab., *11* (Suppl. 1): 109, 1981) mainly show the cell folded along one of its diameters. Are these aspects documenting that here we have to do with membrane (or whole cell) 'flexibility' or 'pliability'? Is this cell folding sufficient to ensure pore passage?

Dr Skalak has discussed theoretically that the RBC membrane will probably have to tank tread while the cell approachs a pore; thereafter, as the red cell flips over the sharp corner of the pore entrance tank treading might be associated with large membrane extensions, which can end up in rupture (in: Symposium on Recent Developments in Microcirculation Research, Jerusalem, April 1981, Eds.: E. David/G.A. Marcel, Excerpta Medica-Amsterdam: 31).

At the present time we do not know exactly what kind of motion a RBC preforms during the few milliseconds of actual passage through a Nuclepore pore: the pore length (12 microns) probably represents too short a pathway for the full development of membrane tank treading, such as seen in the travelling glass tube. It cannot be ruled out, however, that cell gliding along the pore associated with some wall friction could also occur during actual pore passage. On the other hand, evidence is accumulating to support the view that critical events are taking place in the transition regions both at the entrance into and at the exit from the pore: see for example stereoscan electron micrographs by Lessin (Blood Cells, 1977, 3/2: 241–262). At this level adhesion phenomena might also come into play.

Whatever way these complex and intricate phenomena will be described in detail, we are seemingly all coming to agree that *conventional* 'Nuclepore filtrability'* primarily reflects the extent of pore clogging. An individual red cell is either able to pass through a Nuclepore 'pore' or it is not, and thence will obstruct it: an 'all-or-none' phenomenon which most likely can follow from different mechanisms, occurring isolated or in association. As a result, the flow rate through the whole filter will decrease (constant pressure approach) or the filter resistance will increase (constant flow approach).

Coming to the discussion of the paper filters. I would like to make a short introductory comment.

By and large, with any kind of filter system one is endeavouring to simulate in some experimental model 'extra vivum' the geometric and fluid dynamic conditions of the living microcirculation, and this to the best possible extent. A careful scrutiny of different models available discloses this simulation to have been achieved more or less realistically. Before elaborating on particulars, we would first have to clarify several immediate pertinent questions. First: is it actually possible to simulate *all conditions at the same time* and this in a single system? It is my feeling that the appropriate answer is negative. Second question: in this case, what set of conditions should be considered most important and given precedence? Since there appears to be no final answer to this question as yet, the most reasonable approach is to continue making studies with several methods in parallel.

Since their introduction in haemorheological research, Nuclepore filters have been considered as the best available *geometric* models of the capillaries. Attractiveness of their stereoscan electron micrographs and good geometric definition of the pores have been decisive for their rapid and widespread acceptance and utilization. In the process, however, the fluid dynamic conditions in these filters have been overlooked, probably because of their more abstract character. By the same token, geometric and fluid dynamic conditions in the transition regions of entry and exit, as well as the locally corresponding flow patterns and motions of RBC have not received the whole due attention.

Different from Nuclepore sieves, paper filters, Millipore sieves, membranes made of sintered granules and fiber fabrics have irregular, long, tortuous and branched 'equivalent microscopical tubes' (EMT). With these systems we most obviously cannot know the real diameters of the EMT, their variation across the filter, the frequency distribution of EMT diameters in the plane of entry surface

* Systematic utilization of this term will probably be necessary.

(and also in the different planes parallel to it within the filter) and finally their density. While the exact geometric definition of one individual EMT cannot be given for the paper filters, it is nonetheless possible to obtain reliable information on statistically averaged values for the filter membrane as a whole.

These poorly defined geometric parameters notwithstanding, I would like to make a case here for this type of filter and suggest that they might present some positive aspects which probably warrant their reconsideration.

As outlined in a previous publication (Blood Cells, 1977, *3*: 55), polymicroviscometry essentially consists of a continuous monitoring of the decrease in flow rate of *concentrated* red cell suspensions through paper filter as a function of steadily decreasing driving pressures.

But a haematocrit over 70% is also quite an unrealistic simulation of a physiological situation: extreme crowding of red cells is a highly abnormal situation, occurring *in vivo* only in conditions of *considerable flow retardation*. For a long time it has also been my feeling that at least with respect to shear stresses and shear rates, the worst possible flow conditions which can occur *in vivo* (i.e. those near to the point of flow stagnation or 'rheological occlusion'*) are simulated fairly well in the PMV approach. I had, considerable difficulties however, in giving an appropriate answer to the question as to what extent the geometric conditions of the living circulation are also simulated by this type of filter. After all, perhaps this question had to be formulated in some other way, namely in terms of simulating a *critical flow situation* in which the most salient feature of the RBC flow behaviour is challenged.

I would like to submit the proposition that the critical situation best simulated in this type of filters corresponds to that obtaining at the level of a flow divider or vascular branching point. In this situation, it is not an actual RBC 'shape deformation' which is mimicked, but rather a flow pattern and in the first place the specific type of RBC *motion in flow*: membrane tank treading.

A typical critical situation for RBC flowing through an irregular meshwork of fibers is somehow analogous to that shown in Dr Schmid-Schönbein's film to occur *in vivo* at the branching point of a capillary. Different, however, from the real situation *in vivo*, *dense cell crowding* in the EMT of the filter will prevent the one particular red cell straddling on the flow divider to evade from this position in direction of the lumen axis; hence, in order to flow past this point in either one direction this cell will mandatorily have to tank tread. Such a situation is likely to be met repeatedly by the packed RBC as they slowly flow through the paper filter. The thicker the filter, the greater also the number of these flow dividers, where fully developed tank treading is an absolute requirement.

Although relevant evidence is not available, the possibility should also be

* Rheological occlusion of the filter in the PMV approach is different from actual pore occlusion (as in Nuclepore membranes), since diameters of EMT are considerably greater than those of RBC.

considered that tank treading of individual cells likewise will be critically challenged as the packed RBC flow through regions of constrictions or confluence of the EMT.

A complete theoretical analysis of flow patterns and RBC motions through the paper filters cannot be done, since the irregular meshwork of fibers defies any exact geometrical description. Along this line we hope nonetheless, not before long to be in a better position with filters made of sintered granules and/or fiber fabrics which we are presently testing for the PMV approach.

B. *A Stereoscan-electron microscopic study of RBC filtration through different types of filters by H.G. Roggenkamp and P. Teitel**

Figure 4.1, panels A, B and C show the entry, i.e. smooth surface of *control* polycarbonate Nuclepore membranes at the magnifications of 100, 300 and 1600 diameters, respectively. On these micrographs we have to point out the following features: 1) there is an irregular, random distribution of pore entrances; 2) many pores appear to be obstructed by some residual material; 3) some pores are not perfectly perpendicular to the membrane surface, i.e. have lengths greater than the membrane thickness, and 4) a relatively great number of *double pores* can be observed. These aspects strongly suggest that washing and calibration of the membranes prior to their utilization should, by no means, be neglected. The frequency of double pores, through which a RBC will probably not have too much difficulty to pass cannot, however, be derived from a calibration procedure; the only recommendation that can be made in this connection is to utilize membranes with a relatively low pore density. In our hands, the 'Haemaphil'® Nuclepore membranes specially selected for RBC filterability studies did not present aspects of significant better quality.

The 'deformation' of a RBC as it enters into a Nuclepore 'pore' should probably be termed adequately as a *folding* of the whole cell about one of its diameters, which then appears parallel to the pore centreline (Fig. 4.2, panel A). Inside the pore (Fig. 4.2, panel B) the RBC likewise appears 'folded'. As emphasized also by Cokelet (Sand. J. Clin. Lab. Invest., 1981, Suppl. 156 to vol. 41; 77) the kind and extent of membrane 'distortion' under these circumstances seems undefined and unanalyzed. We do not know whether this 'folding' alone is sufficient for actual pore passage.

In some batches of Nuclepore filters the pore diameters do not appear uniform along their length. Aspects of the rough discharge surface of these membranes in

* We acknowledge with thanks the support and cooperation of Dr H.G. Hollweg and Mrs S. Gülpen from the Pathological Institute (Director: Prof Dr Chr. Mittermayer) of the Medical Faculty, RWTH-Aachen.

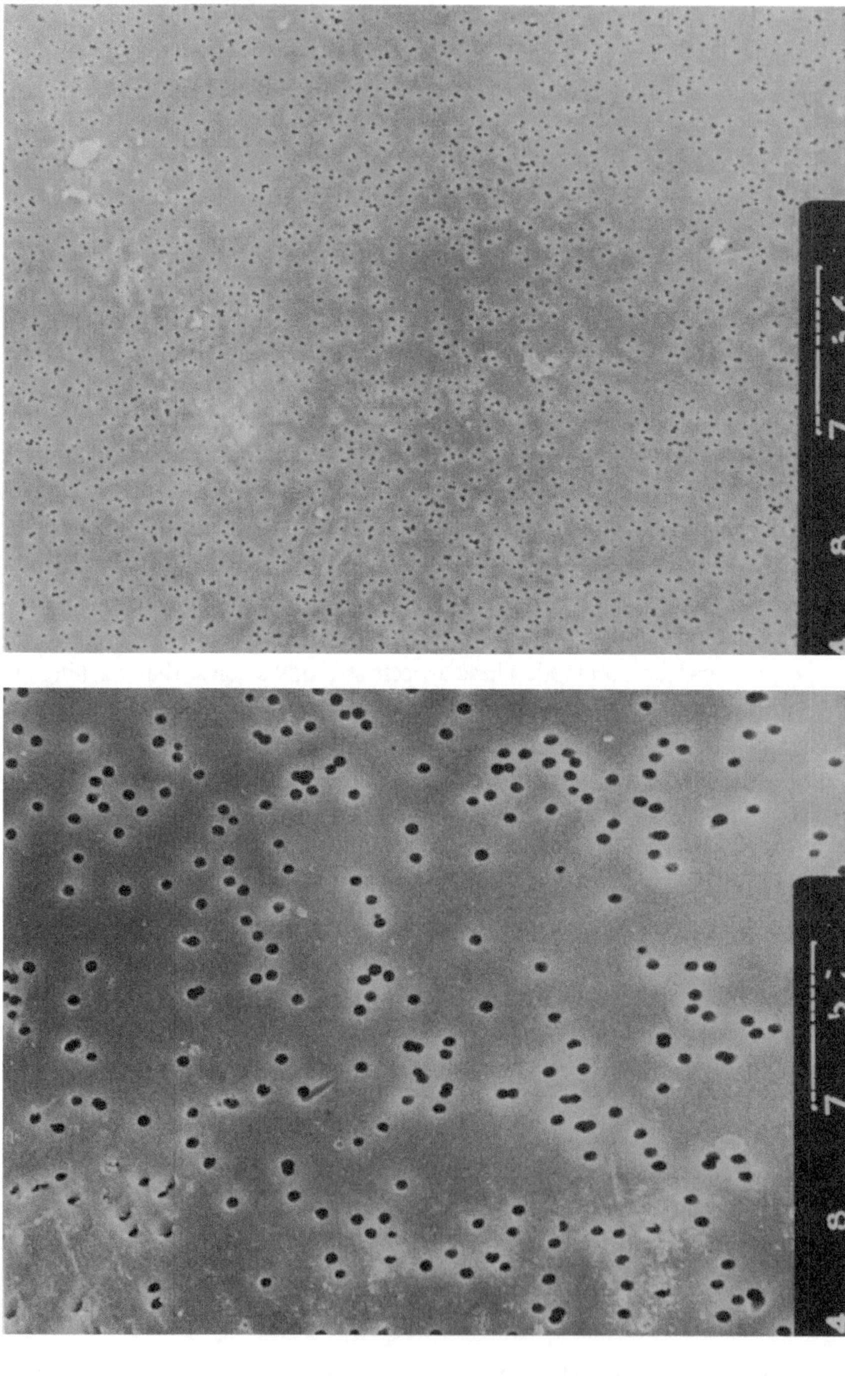

Fig. 4.1 A and B

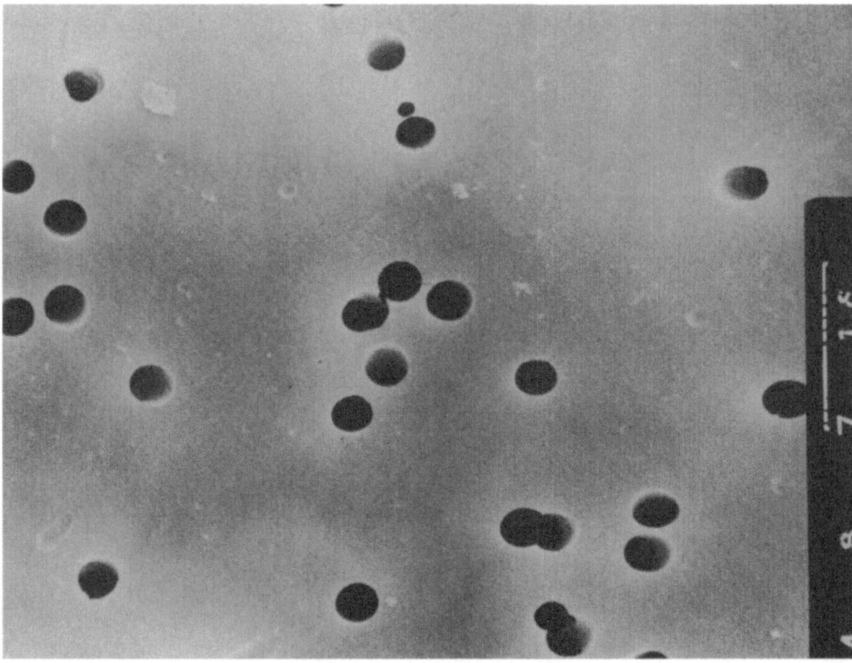

Fig. 4.1 C

the three panels of Fig. 4.3 show frequent *confluent* pore openings greater in diameter than the RBC. Some pores even contain several red cells of normal shape. In addition, the inner walls of some pores (Fig. 4.3, panel C) also present a rough surface. Of course there is always a certain bias in selecting micrographs to be presented; the point I would like to make here is that these aspects suggest it to be desirable to check each membrane batch with the stereoscan electron microscope and discard those presenting such features.

Even with the low hydrostatic pressure head in the Filtrometer, the initial shear stress at the wall of a Nuclepore 'pore' of 5 μm in diameter amounts to approx. 300 dynes/cm^2 (30 Pa); this value seems to be high enough to damage some of the RBC during pore passage, as documented by micrographs from Fig. 4.4. It is very difficult to state whether the corresponding pores will actually be clogged. Some aspects in these micrographs, in which RBC membranes appear as if they were adherent to the pore walls suggest the occurrence of interactions between filter material and RBC. In panel C of Fig. 4.4 the RBC damage seems to result from the interaction with a platelet still present in the RBC suspension in spite of removal of plasma and buffy coat. The probability is small that these aspects of RBC 'damage' are artifacts resulting from glutaraldehyde fixation, since they were absent in all preparations made with the other three types of

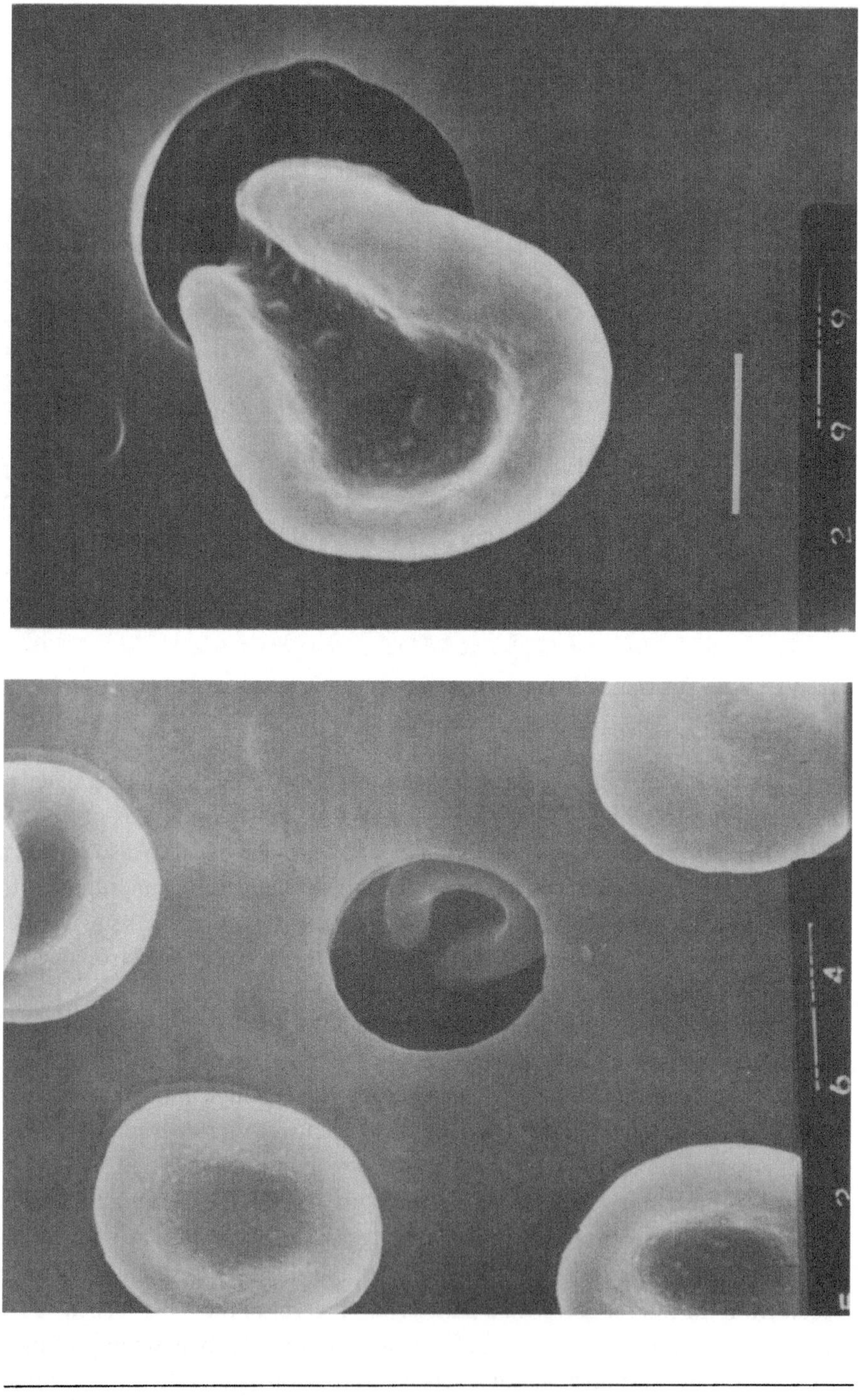

Fig. 4.2 A and B

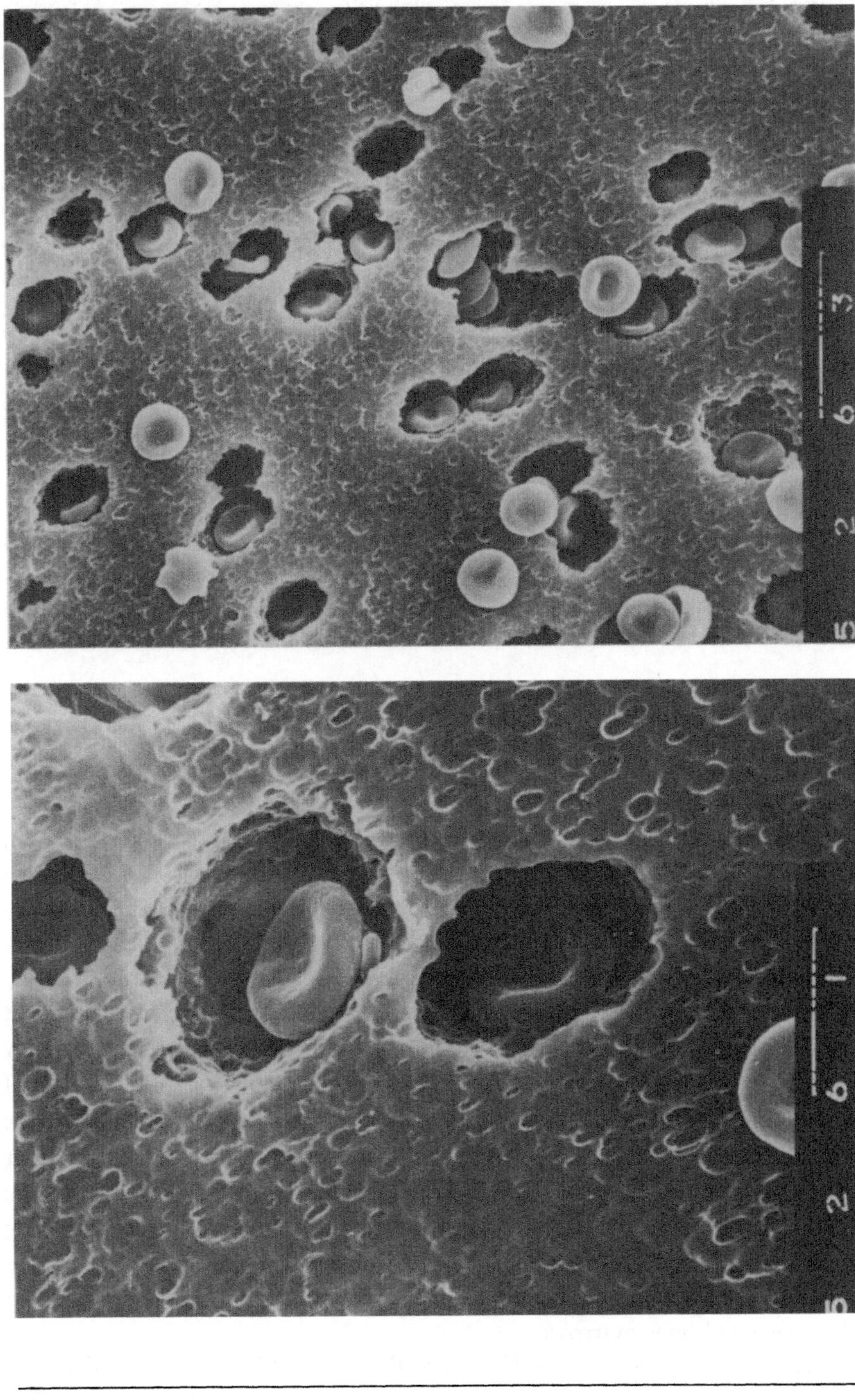

Fig. 4.3 A and B

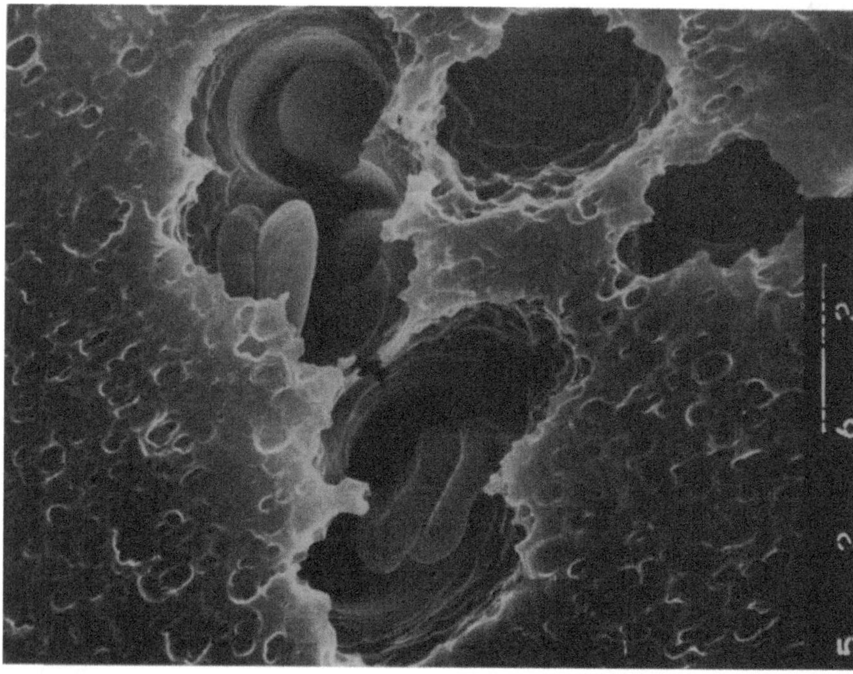

Fig. 4.3 C

filters (which have been fixed exactly the same way).

We linked great hopes to the advent of the metal microprecision sieves, but have been very disappointed by results obtained with these filters; both reproducibility and sensitivity to detect rheological abnormalities of experimentally 'rigidified' RBC could not match those of Nuclepore filters.

Millipore filters still used by a few groups have a 'sponge'-like structure (Fig. 4.5, panels A, B and C) and irregular, long, tortuous and branched 'equivalent microscopic tubes' (EMT) which cannot be defined geometrically. Overview aspects of the entry surface of Millipore filters with a nominal 'pore' diameter of 12 μm (panels D, E and F) suggest that the passage of a RBC through such a complex filter implies a type of 'deformation' different from a mere folding, for which the term 'flow' seems to be more appropriate. In these micrographs, the RBC actually *seem to flow* past the filter structures, frequently leaving a long 'tail' behind them and assuming the most diverse shapes. These aspects are reminiscent of the stereoscan electron micrographs of RBC circulating through the spleen and bone marrow.

According to producer specifications, the usual cellulose nitrate Millipore filters have the property to bind small amounts of protein (and nucleic acids). We

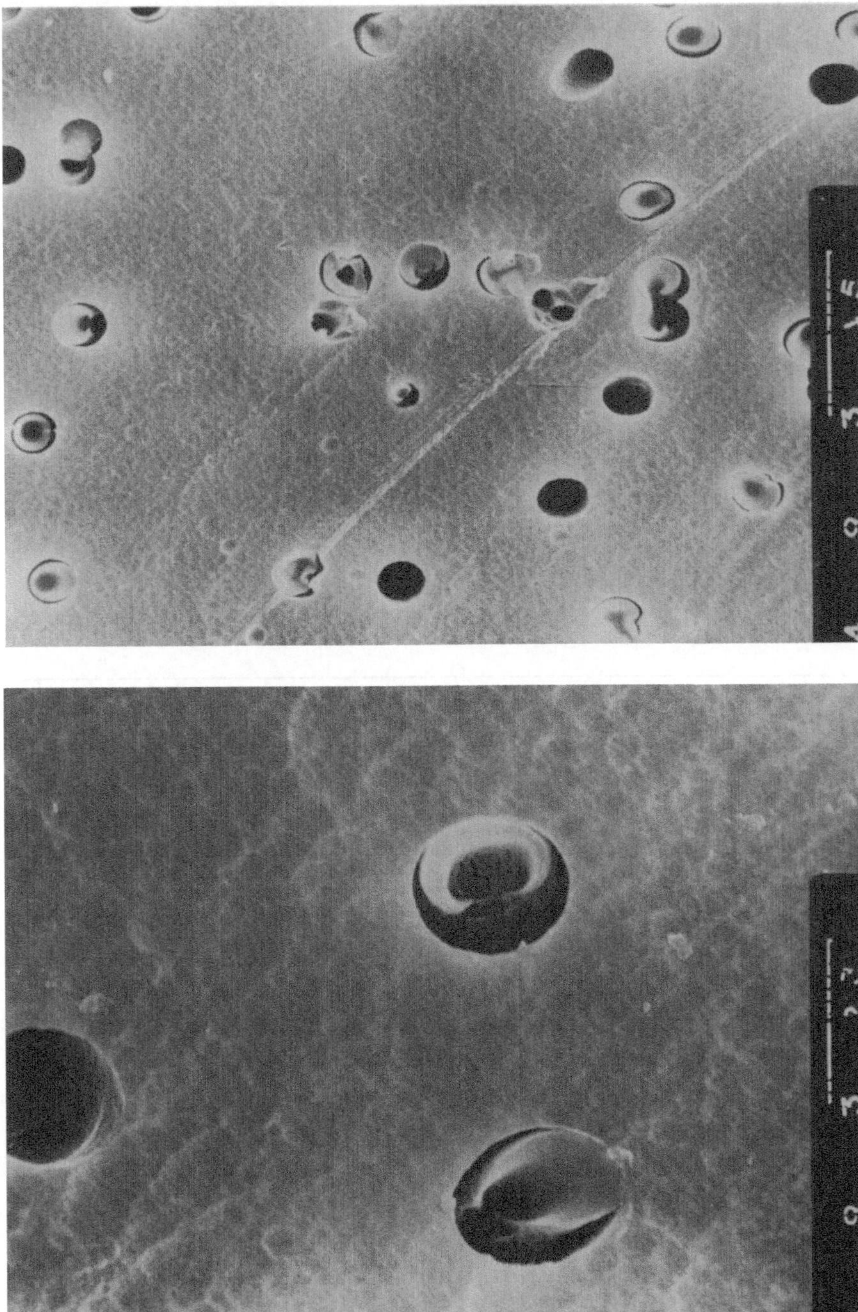

Fig. 4.4 A and B

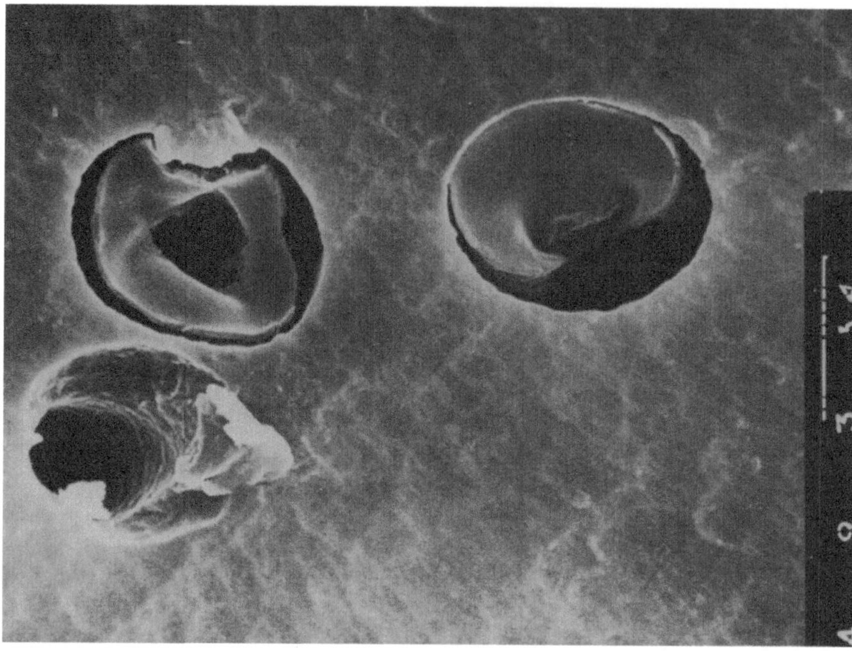

Fig. 4.4 C

could frequently observe aspects (Fig. 4.6, panels A and B) showing punctiform attachment sites of the RBC membranes to the filter material, probably mediated by residual plasma proteins remaining adsorbed onto the RBC membrane even after the three washings with saline. Such kind of attachment could lead to retention of RBC within the filter structure by a mechanism which has nothing to do with rheological behaviour or RBC 'deformability'. Even if no such firm attachment of the RBC to the Millipore filter occurs, the affinity of the cellulose nitrate for proteins could possibly lead also to some changes (in the three-dimensional configuration of constituents or in electrical charge distribution, etc.) at the external face of the RBC membrane, resulting in the tendency to stomatocytosis illustrated in panel C of Fig. 4.6. It cannot be excluded that phenomena of this kind have to be made responsible for the discrepancy of results obtained by Dr Ehrly when comparing the effects of different anticoagulants on Millipore filterability.

I finally turn to the paper filters I have been utilizing for a good number of years now.

Figure 4.7 shows the overview aspect of a paper filter Schwarzband (black ribbon) Nr. 589[1] (Schleicher & Schull) at a magnification of 100 diameters. At the uppermost level of the filter the very first layer of cellulose fibers makes up

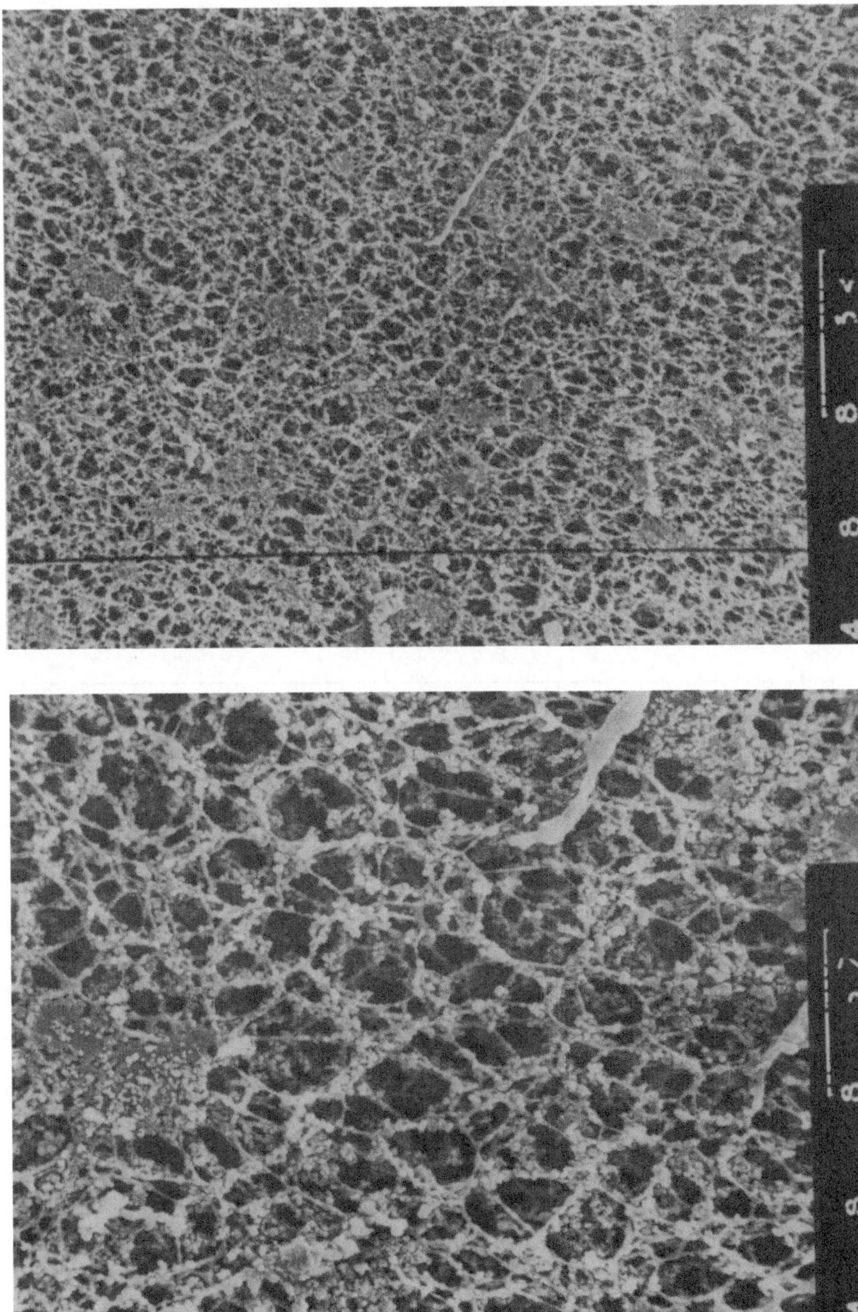

Fig. 4.5 A and B

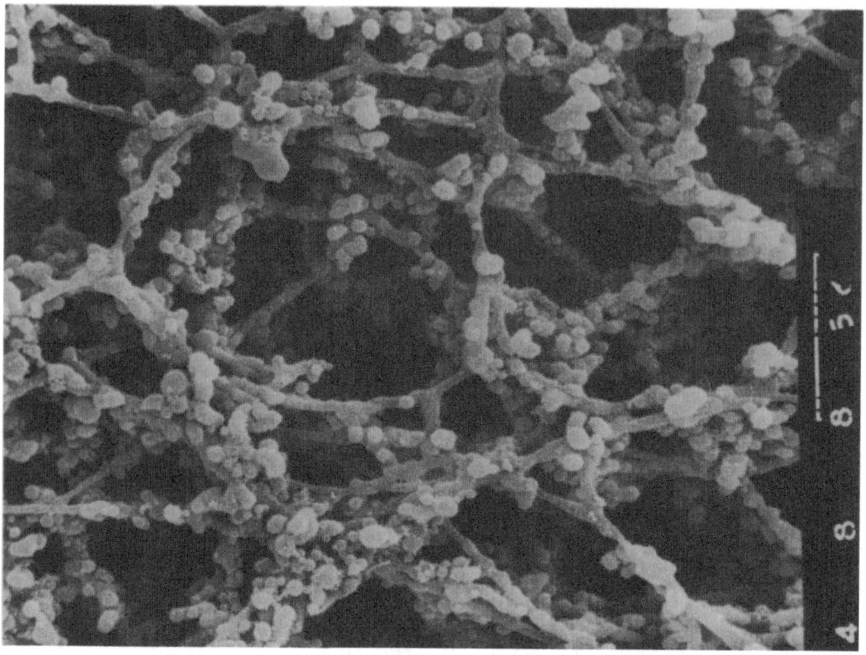

Fig. 4.5 C

only a few percents of the total surface, so that the geometric transient at the filter entrance is initially small and then gradually increases as we penetrate deeper into the filter. Assuming an estimated average fiber diameter of 15–25 μm (see Fig. 4.8), we will have in a filter 800 μm thick a number of 40 superposed parallel layers of fibers similar to that shown on Fig. 4.7. It is obvious that in such a pad of layers there are no real direct channels going from one side to the other of the filter, but again irregular, long, tortuous, branched and confluend 'equivalent microscopic tubes' (EMT) corresponding to the void spaces between the fibers.

Overview micrographs from the four panels in Fig. 4.8 (magnification of 300, 600, 1000 and 2000 diameters, respectively) illustrate the dimensional relationship between RBC, cellulose fibers and void spaces in this type of paper filter. These specimens have been prepared without deep freezing and a great number of RBC have diffused out of the filter during fixation in glutaraldehyde; therefore, these micrographs do not document the real RBC crowding in the void spaces of the filter. No aspects suggesting that RBC membranes are attached to or adsorbed onto the surface of the cellulose fibers are to be seen in these (and numerous others not shown) micrographs. One can also observe that the fibers have no sharp edges (such as always present at the entrance into a Nuclepore pore) but round contours.

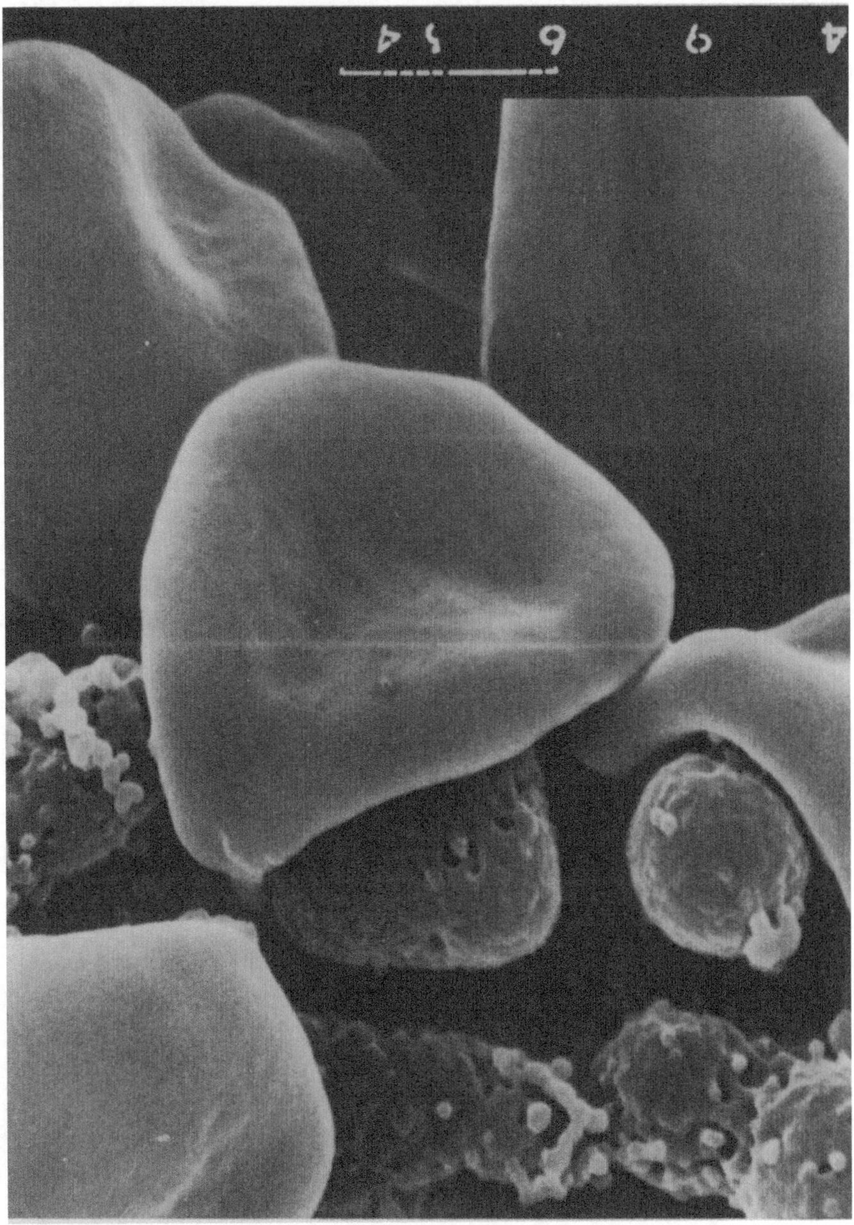

Fig. 4.5 D

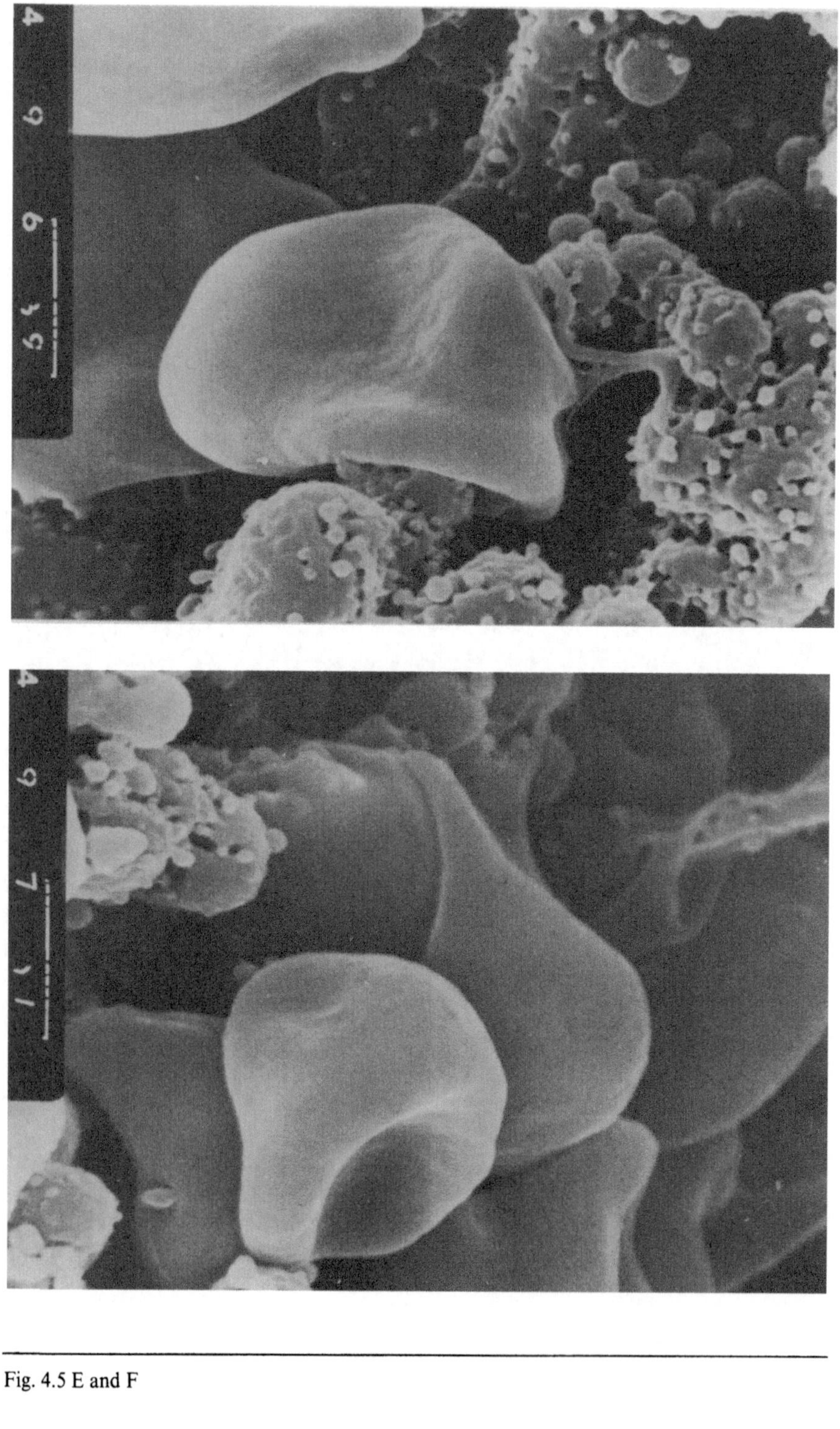

Fig. 4.5 E and F

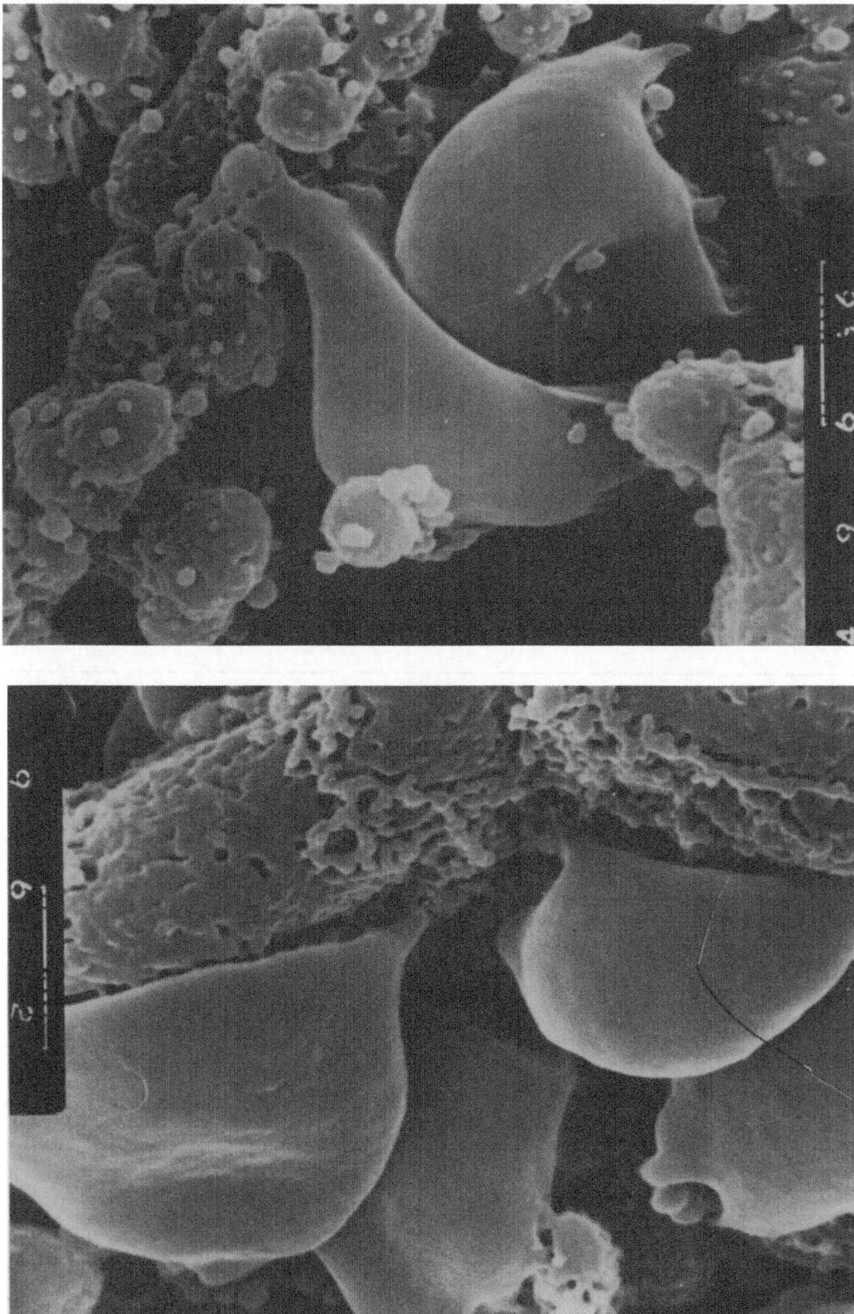

Fig. 4.6 A and B

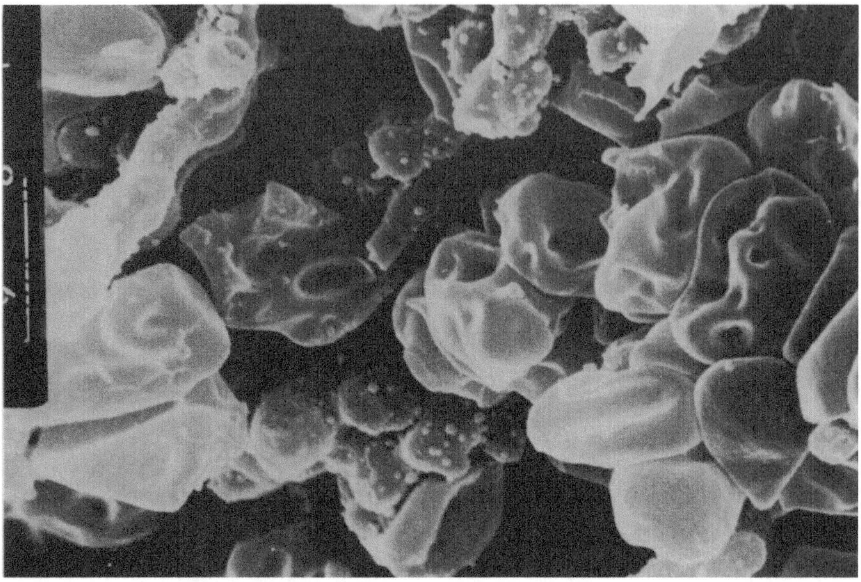

Fig. 4.6 C

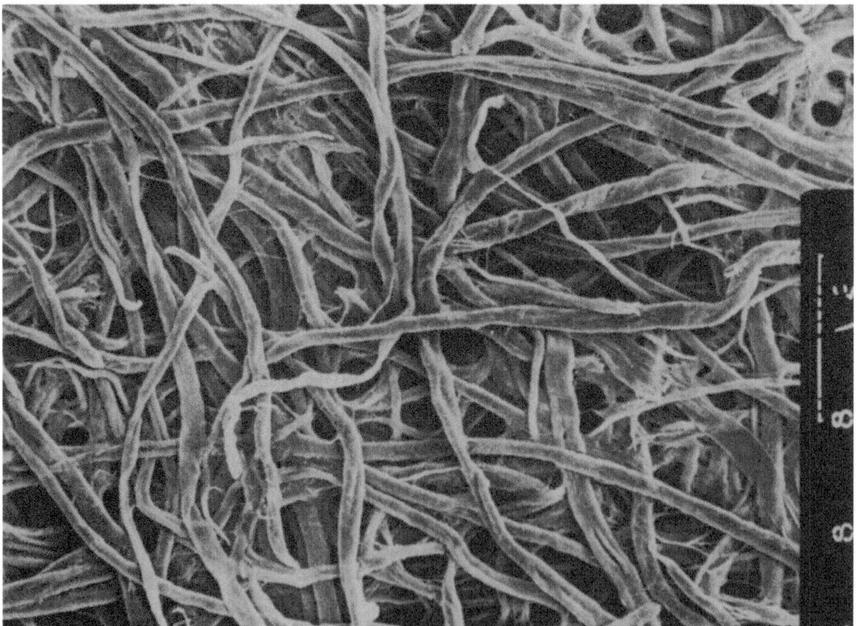

Fig. 4.7

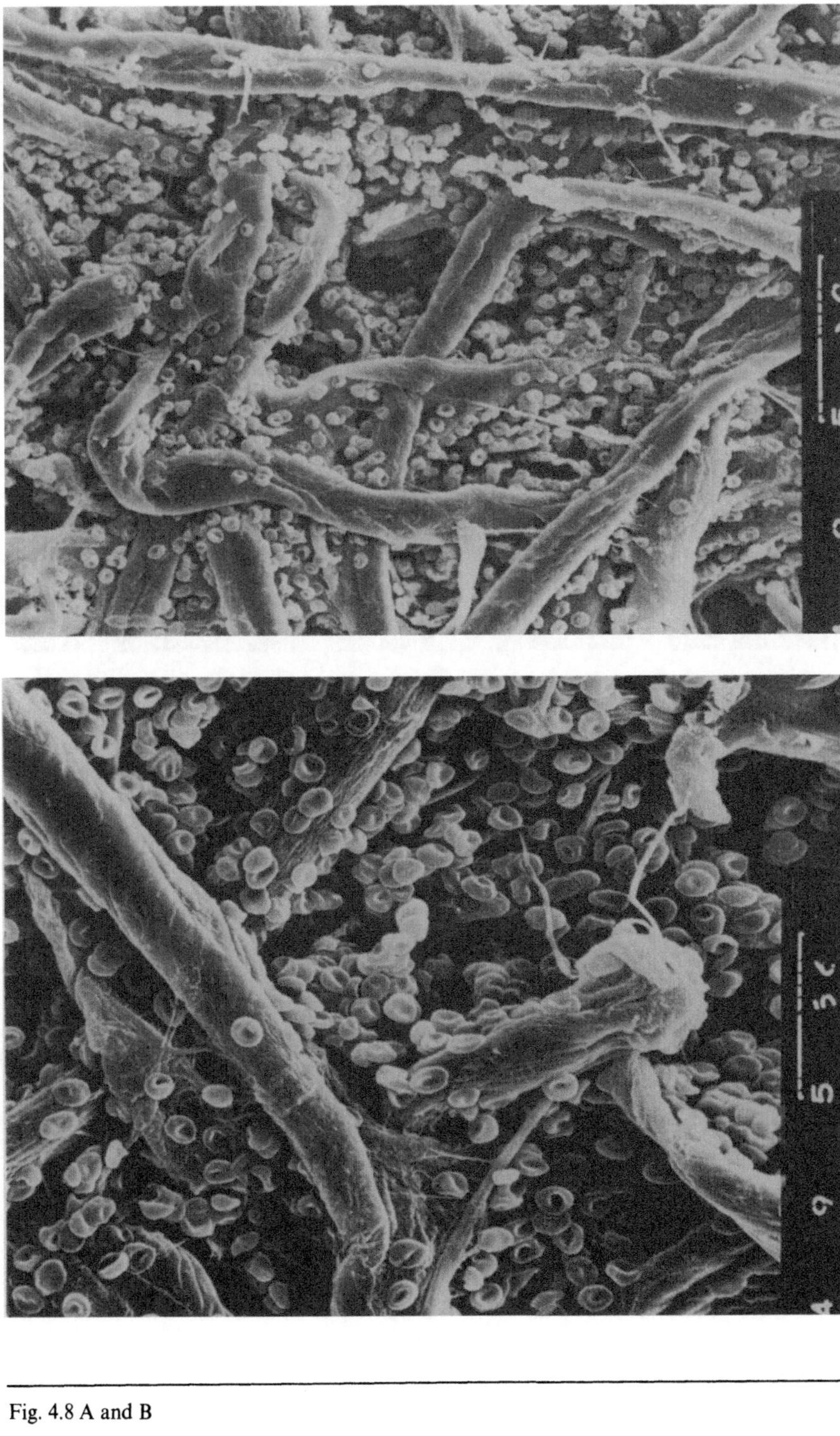

Fig. 4.8 A and B

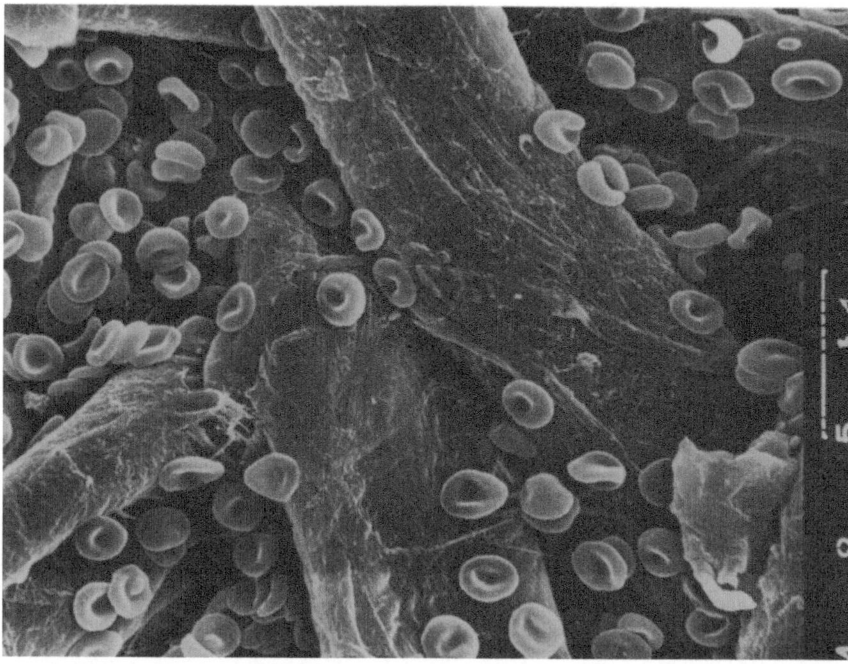

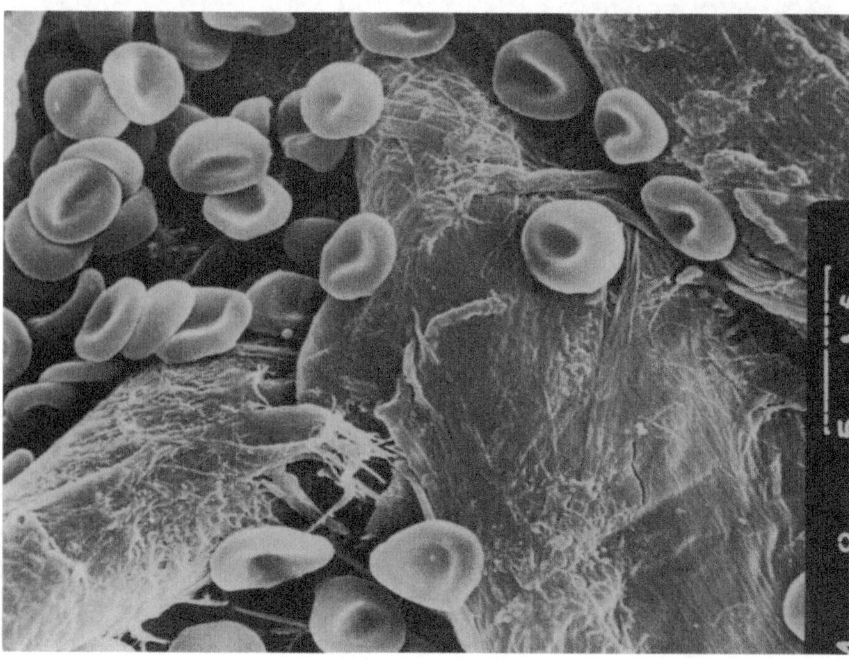

Fig. 4.8 C and D

The most relevant morphologic evidence for *the way RBC are moving* when passing through this type of filter has been obtained in micrographs of freeze-fractured preparations. Figure 4.9 shows the fractured brim of a filter without RBC (panel A: magnification 100 diameters) and with RBC (panel B: magnification 300 diameters). While in the first panel one can see that the ruptured fibers look like the bristles of a brush, in the second one the following features are obvious: 1) at the entrance into the filter (upper part) the densely crowded RBC forming sort of a pancake and 2) in the filter interior, the fibers which have been torn away (with the other fracture fragment) leave behind them their imprint in the RBC 'pancake'. The four panels in Fig. 4.10 (magnification of 1000, 24000, 3000 and 7500 diameters, respectively) show blow ups of such a fiber imprint'. In panels A and B one can see the cast of RBC around the fiber which has been pulled out from the specimen while fracturing the filter membrane and the 'deformation' of the red cells resulting from both interaction between one another and also interaction with the fiber. At the greater enlargements of the panels C and D the polygonal aspect of the packed RBC in close contact with a fiber can better be seen.

Thank you very much for your attention.

P.G. Thank you Dr Teitel. Any specific questions or comments related to these presentation?

J.S. In a sectional drawing or micrograph of a Nuclepore pore we always see a right angle edge at the entrance, with a sharp contour which is totally unphysiological. Is the damage to the cell membrane produced mechanically as the cell flips over this edge? Is there also an interaction between the red cell membrane and the polycarbonate material in the Nuclepore filters as you suggest that we get with Millipore filters?

P.T. I think that it is primarily a mechanical effect, resulting from this geometry and the fluid dynamic conditions. The micrographs suggest that an interaction with the polycarbonate would occur after production of such a damage.

J.S. And should we design filters with a smoother entrance such as seen with the metal filters?

P.T. I think we should, since entrance effects seem to be critical in conventional Nuclepore filtration. Fabrics of plastic fibers and filters made of sintered spheres are now available and we are presently testing them. In our opinion we have to look for better filters, in which both geometric and fluid dynamic conditions would mimick more closely the conditions prevailing in the microcirculation. The thickness of the uretal filter is ten microns.

H.S-S. The pores in the metal sieves have a cylindrical part of ten microns in length and a cone-shaped entrance on the one face. If RBC enter the filter through the cone-shaped entrances the flow rates are extremely high and it is very difficult to differentiate between a normal and a model abnormal red cell. If I am

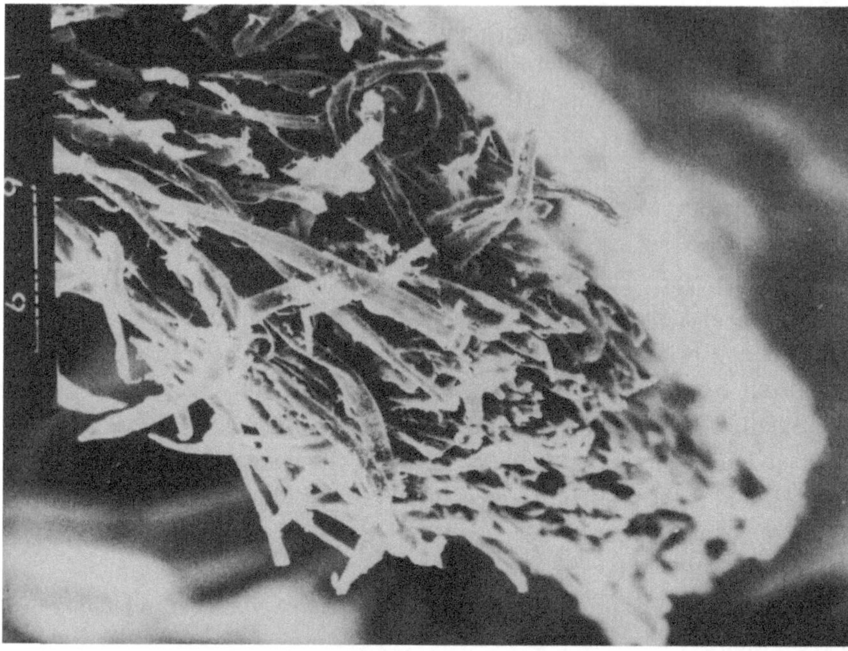

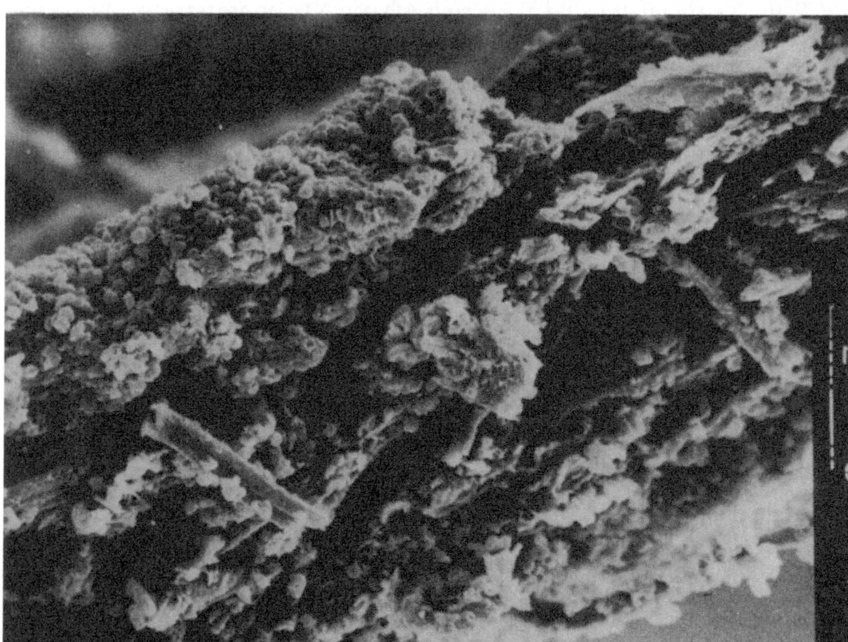

Fig. 4.9 A and B

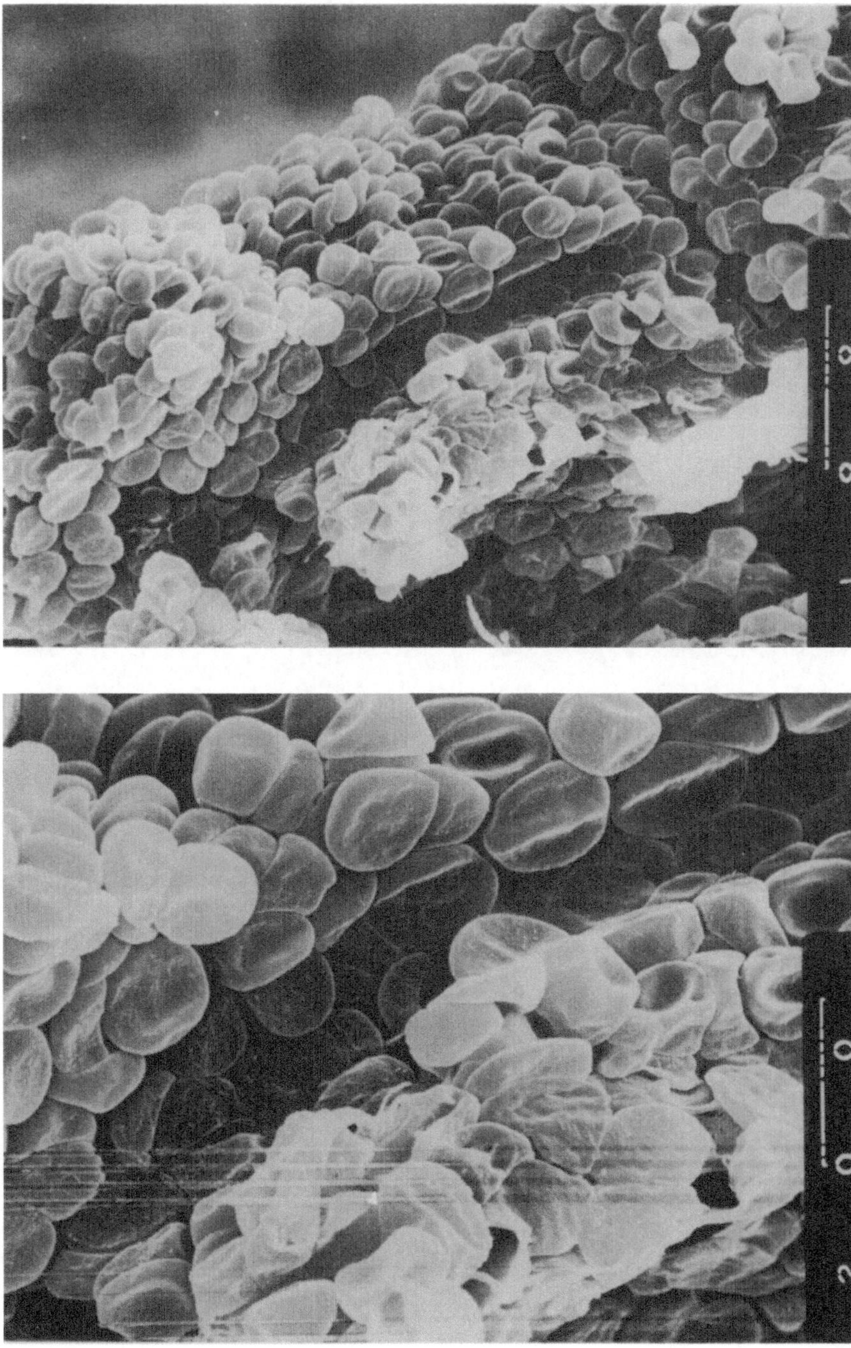

Fig. 4.10 A and B

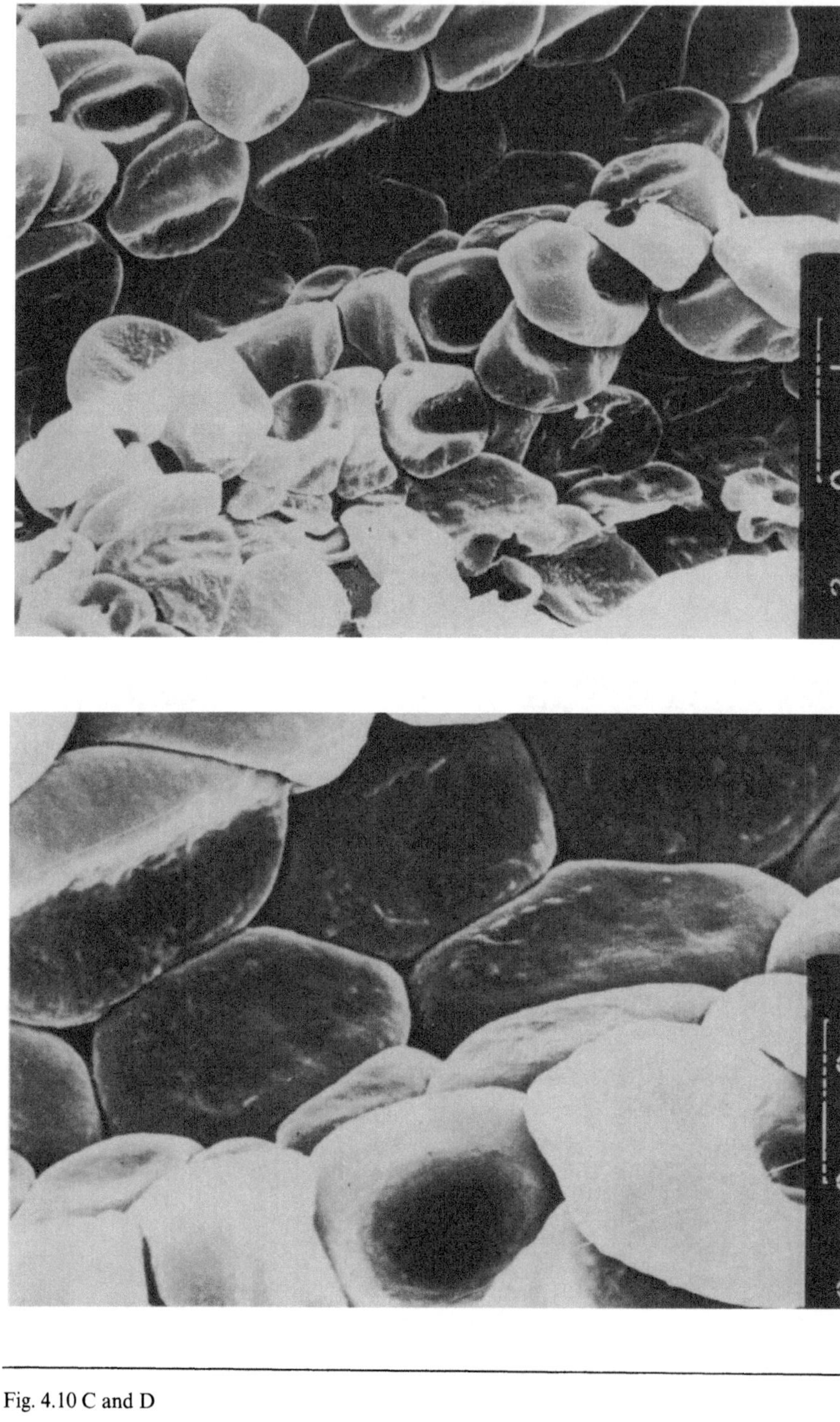

Fig. 4.10 C and D

correct, Dr Stoltz has also made some measurements with these filters and it would be interesting to hear from his experience.

JF.S. We have also used the metal sieves recently and have been confronted with the same kind of difficulties as mentioned by Dr Teitel.

S.C. There are many different kinds of filters which have been used. Historically, the paper filters were the very first ones and they do have their virtues as Dr Teitel has pointed out. Because of their irregularities maybe they simulate certain microcirculatory conditions better than the more straightforward polycarbonate filters, although it is easier to standardise the polycarbonate filters than the paper ones. I agree with Dr Teitel in that a RBC has to fold in order to enter into a Nuclepore pore; we have obtained micrographs showing this as early as 1970. With reference to the question of Dr Stuart we also saw that the corner at the entrance into a Nuclepore pore is relatively sharp: if we use very high pressures, like those Dr Meiselman talked about yesterday, and smaller size filter pores we do get hemolysis at the corners.

The last point I would like to make is that when pores are very close together this may not necessarily facilitate the flow of the cells. Actually, the same cell may try to get into two pores at the same time and get stuck there. It is important, therefore, to avoid these coincidences of pores when we use any type of filter.

P.G. Thank you very much.

J.S. Does anyone know what happens with a RBC as it is going down through a Nuclepore pore 10 microns in length: does it rattle from side to side or does it go straight down the middle with no tank treading?

R.S. I think the possibility of going straight down without any tank treading is very small. To do this a red cell would have to enter perfectly symmetrically into a pore, which is essentially a zero probability. So the answer is: there will be some tank treading.

J.S. How can it tank tread on both sides at the same time?

R.S. It will tend to tank tread on both sides at the same time but in opposite directions.

J.S. Would it not be nice to make a transparent filter so that you could take photographs of this mechanism?

R.S. I think it has been done; it is called intravital microscopy.

P.G. But not on such short channels of approx. 13 microns in length.

R.S. Yes, I agree that it would be nice to actually see what happens with a red cell as it goes through a pore in the filter.

H.S-S. A short comment. I am of course convinced that tank treading plays an important role in the rheological behaviour of red cells. I would like to emphasize the fact that at the moment it is still undecided whether Nuclepore filterability is governed by entrance effects or passage effects. I have very strong feelings about the necessity to analyse entrance phenomena, since we see that a single filter changes its hydraulic conductivity during a measurement especially when working with a pathological sample. this indicates that red cells have greater problems to enter into a 5 micron pore rather than to pass through it.

P.G. Thank you very much. That will now end this session and we will move on to the next one.

SESSION 5

Filtration equipment

In this session four filtration methods were presented on videotape by Drs Forconi, Hanss, Marcel and Stoltz. An edited videotape of these four presentations (length 30 minutes, VFS system) is available from Dr George Szendey, Hoechst AG, Pharmaceutical Division, Verkauf Pharma Ausland – ZPM, 6230 Frankfurt/Main, West Germany.

S.F. In Siena, a modification of the red cell filtration method described by Reid, Dormandy and colleagues is used. Whole blood is filtered through a 5 μ pore diameter Nuclepore filter under a negative pressure of 20 cm water. The major modification is that the syringe containing the sample and the filter holder are surrounded by a 37° C water jacket, to ensure that the measurements are conducted at 37°. Freshly-drawn anticoagulated whole blood is kept at 37° C prior to measurement. The volume of red cells filtered per minute is calculated from the measured filtration time and from the haematocrit. Comparative studies at 22° C, 30° C and 37° C show the most reproducible results at 37° C. In Siena, much importance is given to the correct temperature for serving the local Chianti wine. All the more reason therefore to ensure the correct temperature for filtration of blood.

A videotape of the method used by S. Forconi followed.

J.S. How could you guarantee that you do not get water leakage into your blood system, from your water jacket, and you get haemolysis? How can you guarantee the seal when you plug it?

S.F. No, it is very simple with a silicone cap. There is definitely no water. No haemolysis.

P.L. Just a very short comment I made yesterday. I suggest that the temperature difference is mostly due to the effect of temperature on white blood cells more than on red cells.

S.F. Yes, I will comment. We studied some patients with leukocytosis and some isolated examples of patients with chronic myeloid leukemia. In our method there is not any clear influence of the white cells, even when their number increases. The filtration index gets worse only in presence of a very high number and in presence of a high percentage of blasts, but not when only normal granulocytes have increased. We have the opinion that the white cell number, in the range we normally measure, does not influence V_{RBC}, if we take measurements immediately after the withdrawal, at 37° C, with a slight anticoagulant excess. Can the influence of white cells possibly be greater if we measure at room temperature and after storage of blood?

J.D. Can I just follow that up? Using this technique, which is quite unique in that you make your measurements immediately, at body temperature, and you remove nothing, you have found very interesting clinical results. Have you tried to correlate your RCF with the white cell count of the patient? What is the correlation between the white cell count of the patient and the filtration value which you obtain 60 seconds or 2 minutes later?

S.F. No correlation.

J.S. May I come back to the point that Pierre Leblond made just now. You say that if you filter whole blood there is an obvious temperature dependence. (Yes). The ideal experiment would be to filter blood with the leukocytes and the platelets removed to see if temperature dependence is still present, but you have not done that yet? (No). You did say that you did look at the blood from a leukaemic patient with a very high white cell count. (Yes). Is the temperature dependence of that blood still present?

S.F. I don't know. We did only single measurements on chronic leukaemic patients and, as on other patients, always at 37°. We have only an impression that a considerable amount of white blood cells does not affect the measurements, but we have only a few cases, not sufficient for a definite answer.

S.C. Did you measure the effect of temperature on the filtration of plasma?

S.F. No.

M.H. It is a question maybe for Shu Chien. Do you have evidence that the white blood cells have the same rigidity as red blood cells when you have the same experimental procedure? In other words, are all experiments with white blood cells which are supposed to block all the pores artefacts due to low temperature conservation of the blood prior to measurement?

S.C. We have studied the deformability of the red cells versus white cells with the micropipette technique. In terms of the steady state behaviour, white cells are about five times as rigid as red cells. In terms of the dynamic behaviour, the viscosity parameter, the white cells are about 1000 times more viscous than the red cells. At 37° as well as at room temperature.

P.L. I think Marshall Lichtman once also did measurements on white cells with micropipettes and he did show, at least for granulocytes, that temperature had a profound effect on the behaviour of such white cells in micropipettes.

S.C. Yes, I agree. We recently published a paper in *Biophysical Journal* by Sung *et al* and indeed it shows that even with small deformations, Lichtman did large deformations, we did small deformations and showed the same thing.

J.S. May I repeat the plea that was made yesterday that when we talk about white cells we begin to define what we mean. When you talk about white cells and Lichtman's work are you talking about neutrophil polymorphs, lymphocytes, or monocytes?

P.L. I was referring to granulocytes of different maturation stages, which is what he had published.

S.C. The paper that I referred to, the two papers published in the *Biophysical Journal* were on neutrophils. Recently we have had some data on lymphocytes; using the micropipette technique with small deformation, their behaviour is very similar. However we did not do the whole cell deformation. I think the lymphocytes are a little smaller than the neutrophils so they may have an easier time to get through the polycarbonate filters.

S.F. I think also that we have no effect from white cells because of the very high shear stress that we use. In these conditions, non-physiological shear stress, the effect of granulocytes in minimised.

P.G. If it is true what Pierre Leblond said yesterday, it does not really matter how many white cells you have in there because even the smallest number of white cells will upset the measurement. So you might not even expect a correlation with white cell count if you go up to 100,000 (pers. comm.). Because if only 50 do it, you do not need 100,000. You will not notice the difference. I am sure that we will come back to this point over and over again. Let us move to the next video which is Dr Hanss'.

M.H. The 'Hemorheometre' is an instrument based on the initial flow rate measurement of a diluted red blood cell (RBC) suspension through a polycarbonate Nuclepore filter (diameter 13 mm, pore diameter 5 μ). The driving force is the hydrostatic pressure (about 5 cm H_2O) given by the vertical liquid column. The top air-liquid interface activates two optoelectronic level sensors D_1 and D_2 separated from each other by about 8 mm (see Fig. 1.6). The electric signals given by these sensors start, then stop an electronic chronometer. The time lapse given by the chronometer is proportional to the flow rate, which is proportional to the apparent fluidity of the liquid being filtered. When this liquid is the suspension, a time lapse t_g is obtained; for the suspending medium (solvent) the time lapse will be called t_s. The total volume of the glass tubing shown is about 1 ml; the volume flow corresponding to the time lapse is about 500 μl. Therefore, as a first order of approximation, the time lapse is proportional to the initial flow rate. A filterability index, IF, is defined as follows:

$$IF = \frac{t_g - t_s}{t_s} \quad \frac{100}{H}$$

where H is the haematocrit (in %). High IFs indicate low RBC filterability. In order to measure IF, the membrane is first calibrated by measuring t_s; then, without changing or moving the membrane, t_g is measured. In our apparatus for H = 8% and normal RBCs, t_s is about 0.5 sec and t_g about 0.8 sec. For a given suspension, the reproducibility is about ± 1% for t_s and ± 3% for t_g.

The suspension is prepared by centrifugation of the anticoagulated blood (500 g, 10 min) and gentle aspiration of 0.4 ml of the middle part of the packed cells. The cells are resuspended in 10^{-2} M Tris-HCl buffered isotonic saline (pH 7,40) with the addition of: KCl: 4 mmol · l^{-1}; glucose: 5.5 mmol · l^{-1}; human serum albumin: 0.5 g · l^{-1}. This solvent is always filtered (Millipore 0.45 μ) prior to the preparation of the suspension.

As previously defined, the filterability index is essentially independent of the filter characteristics. However, membranes with high pore coincidences should be avoided. Therefore, in a particular batch, the membranes with low flow resistance (as measured by t_s) are eliminated.

In the course of at least 500 examinations, we have measured the RBC filtration on EDTA- and heparin-anticoagulated samples taken from a donor or a patient at the same time. We have always found that the RBC in the EDTA-anticoagulated samples had higher IFs (more rigid) than the heparin-anticoagulated samples. Also, the results are more regular with the heparin samples. The filtration index IF takes into account the haematocrit. It has been shown by Healy's group that, as defined previously, IF is independent of H for values lower than 10%.

The advantages of the 'Hemorheometre' may be summarised as follows:

1. The measurements are easy, fast (a few minutes), and precise (electronic chronometer).
2. The membrane hydraulic conductance is measured for each sample so that, as a first order approximation, the filtration index is membrane-independent.
3. The same membrane can be used many times.
4. The initial flow rate principle and the use of a diluted RBC suspension eliminate significantly the adverse effect of the membrane clogging.
5. Once the suspension has been introduced into the measuring chamber, the measurement is finished a few seconds later. Therefore the sedimentation of the RBC over the membrane can be neglected.

A videotape of the method used by M. Hanss followed.

S.C. The suspension filtration time increases progressively in the three tests and you attribute that to the progressive clogging. Now in that case would it not be better to use the first test only?

M.H. We only use the first one, but we systematically do at least three or four measurements in order to be sure that the first one was coherent with the other ones. In some instances the increase is very large from one test to the other. This is probably due to aggregation of red blood cells and this we know because when we make turbulent flow over the membrane with a syringe then the figures go down again.

J.D. I do not want to suggest complicating a beautifully simple machine, but do you not think that if you added a third photoelectric cell so that you could get the flow rate over two intervals then you would get a lot more information in terms of rate of clogging?

M.H. Well, I think the best idea would be to have a continuous flow measuring system and there may be some development with this later. But I do not know whether it is very important because yesterday we heard that it was very complicated to get red blood cell properties out of complete filtration experiments. Because as soon as you have white blood cells then it is very complicated, and as I said in the paper which has been given to everybody, the measurement must be as fast as possible because as soon as the measurement lasts, say, a few tenths of a second then you have complicating factors such as sedimentation over the membrane. So you must do the measurements as fast as possible, and any experiment where the suspension or the blood stays over the membrane for say a minute then the haematocrit over the membrane is much higher than the mean haematocrit.

I.J. We have tried to make ten measurements with the same filter to see if we could have the information of the initial rate and of the plugging, but our results were uninterpretable, not reproducible.

G.A.M. I would like to make a statement to see how people react. This is the only apparatus and method used in more than 10 laboratories throughout the world which could lead to a publication using the words 'red cell deformability'. In other words, if you are on an editorial board and somebody – Holger's questions from yesterday – comes up with a paper saying he has used this machine and this protocol and that he has measured red cell deformability, would you accept the paper for publication?

J.D. Why don't you ask for a show of hands out of interest? (Show of hands).

P.G. The majority say yes.

H.M. I don't believe that there are three numbers coming out within 1% of each other. We discussed yesterday the question of trying to calculate an intrinsic cellular mechanical property by somehow extrapolating back to zero haematocrit. Dick, have you talked about this? Because now that I understand it, it appears that you are basically computing a specific viscosity divided by concentration which seems to be independent of concentration.

R.S. Exactly.

H.M. Which is somewhat surprising. I would have thought there would have been a slope to that line and at the zero intercept, that is at zero haematocrit, in this case there would be an intrinsic value. But it is independent of that from the range of 8 to 0.5% haematocrit. Is that what I understand?

R.S. Yes, and this fits together with the theory we presented and I am prepared to lay that out in a few minutes.

S.C. Just to answer Herb's question quickly. If you plot the ratio against the haematocrit it shows a straight line with a slope and that slope is constant. That is what he is using. That is the slope that is constant. And that is the value he says is constant.

H.S-S. We have had the opportunity to measure with Dr Hanss' instrument. We have chosen 10% haematocrit as a rule, and we have a different way of expressing our data, but in essence the data are identical with one important difference. If you remember in the film we had for the 50 microlitres which are passed through this filter for the saline about 490 msec, and for the red cell suspension about 800 msec, as one goes up to a haematocrit of 10 this comes up to about 1000–1200 msec. Of course, with a very simple calculation one can now calculate the relative flow rate, which in his experiment today on the tape (I just did it) was 0.61. As we have shown repeatedly, using our system in which 1 ml is passed under a much lower pressure and in plasma, we consistently have for normal blood a relative flow rate of 0.65 and after removing all the white cells with a Nacao filter we come up to 0.7. So there is, as I indicated yesterday, a problem of entrance effects. And this becomes more pronounced in this instrument as one reduces the pressure, which we have done very simply by supplying a little extra pressure under the filter. As we go down to the 50 mm of water that we use routinely in the system that I originally devised, we come down to relative flow rates which are in the order of 0.2 to 0.3. Even in saline there is this very important entrance effect, which becomes more important as the cells are rigid and which I think has to be controlled. But this caveat does not keep me from raising my hand and saying that the entrance effect is one aspect of a complex flow behaviour which is obviously often altered in disease. Therefore it is a valid test but we need more analyses of what is going on as these cells enter.

J.S. Tony Marcel asked if we would accept for publication a paper in which it was claimed that this apparatus measured red cell deformability. I was one of the few who responded negatively to that, for three reasons. One, because it is a question of semantics, and provided that the author defined what he means by deformability or filtration and what he is filtering then that is fine by me, whatever words he uses in the title. The second thing is that I would not give a carte blanche acceptance because it could be a lousy paper! And the third thing, the only serious point, is has anyone using the Hanss haemorheometer looked at the effect of white cells in the filtrate on the rate of filtration? In other words has someone deliberately *in vitro* established a range of white cell counts and used the instrument to plot the filtration index against the white cell count in the filtrate? Is the instrument independent of contaminating leukocytes?

M.H. We have not done the measurement which you are asking for, but I am just having a look at the figures which are given on the paper which we have done after all the measurements. There does not seem to be any correlation between the filtration index and the white blood cell count in the suspension.

A.E. I feel the same as Dr Stuart in connection with Marcel's question. I have two other reasons. The first one, if I say yes to accept the paper as an editor in this special condition, I would like to have some personal experience. The second is I do not believe that the scientific truth is a question of a majority opinion!

M.H. I feel pretty sure that what we are measuring is directly connected to the individual red blood cell transit time in the pore. So the question is, is that deformability measurement? If yes, then the filtration index is a deformability measurement. If not, it is very complicated, and it is a matter of defining what is deformability. But that is another question, it is not an experimental question, it is not a question of method, it is a question of philosophy. And I would like to reply to Herbert Meiselman about the 2% precision. This is the precision we get on buffer because we have the 50 Hertz as a clock, for the meter. But on the latest apparatus there is an internal clock so that we can have a better precision on buffer.

P.G. Thank you very much. Now I think we should move on to the next video which is Tony Marcel's video.

G.A.M. Things seemed very simple at the end of the first Working Group Meeting last year. One recommended method was to filter diluted blood at a constant flow rate and to interpret the pressure tracing with respect to time, for example by extrapolation to zero time. So that is what we tried to do. The first decisions we had to make were to decide which haematocrit and which shear stress to use. After reviewing the literature, we decided to use a physiological haematocrit (10%) but a non-physiological shear stress (up to 4000 dynes/cm^2). Blood from healthy volunteers was diluted with buffer to a haematocrit of 10%. Buffer was pumped at a constant flow rate through 5 μm pore diameter Nuclepore filters, and pressure across the filter was measured by a pressure transducer and recorded on a strip chart. The diluted blood was then filtered through the same filter and the pressure after one minute was recorded. Results showed that the method appeared to have pharmacological significance, in that filterability was improved by incubation with oxpentifylline (Trental). However in 7 subjects the filtration pressure was correlated with the plasma fibrinogen concentration and with the leucocyte count. Therefore, in the words of the French philosopher, 'riennest simple' – nothing is simple!

A videotape of the method used by G.A. Marcel followed.

P.L. It was not clear to me whether these were washed cells of whole blood?

G.A.M. These were not washed cells. That was using diluted blood o 10% haematocrit.

P.L. And the shear stress that you indicated, it was 4000 dynes/cm^2?

G.A.M. Of course it varied from one measurement to another, but it was usually between 1500 and 4000 dynes/cm^2.

H.M. A technical question. I noticed that the syringe pump that you use is an

American pump? No it is not, that is what I was going to point out. In fact we have used about six in the laboratory and their most notable feature is about 30% variation in volumetric flow rate. That is, the average flow that they deliver is very very good, there are little numbers that you can set and those are extraordinarily accurate if you integrate the flow over a period of five minutes or so. But if you look at instantaneous flow delivered by the pump there is a variation of plus or minus 20–30%, and I wonder if what we might begin to worry about is, are we in fact imposing a cyclical oscillation on top of a steady flow situation?

G.A.M. We found it is a small variation and we saw it on our curves as you have, and we could easily draw a straight line through it.

H.M. What is your estimate of the variation as a percent of the total pressure, let us say for buffer?

G.A.M. Variation due to the screw of the machine? (Yes). I really think that with a ruler and with a pencil we can eliminate it. We have seen it, it is clear, it is very regular, I could not calculate a figure like that but you can draw a line through it. Although I quite agree that it exists and we have had an engineer look at it already.

H.M. There is no hope, as far as I know, for that pump. I spent a lot of time playing with it, and you cannot eliminate that. Perhaps it may be physiological to impose a bit of slow oscillation on it. Was there any haemolysis in your system?

G.A.M. No, we checked for haemolysis with LDH and we found absolutely none. Even at 4000 dynes/cm^2.

G.L. I have two comments, seeing Tony was waving about the report of last year's meeting. Firstly my apologies to all concerned for the quality of that red tracing, which bears no resemblance to anything in real life, as any of you who have filtered will know! Secondly, as regards Tony's title, as the man who wrote the document, I think nowhere do I claim that anything is simple! I think of course no particular method was recommended; what we did suggest was that the results of any test must be interpreted with regard to time. Simply drawing a line is one approach, but as you have shown nicely and as I think all of us agree, drawing lines is simple but it is more complicated than that!

G.A.M. Please Gordon. It was written with great clarity which only led me to think it was simple!

S.C. Tony, in the videotape you gave a rationale for using the 10% haematocrit. I think in the discussion yesterday and today we probably all agree that we try to extract some kind of intrinsic material property of the cell from the filtration data, and therefore you come down to one single cell and the question is whether the haematocrit range that you use allows you to extract such information. And within that range I do not think it really matters, so we do not really have to apologise for using 10% or 5% or 20% haematocrit. As long as we think that we can extract the proper information out of it for the single cell. I think that as regards the living microcirculation you quoted papers on the haematocrit being 10%. I think a lot of that has to do with temporal and spatial fluctuations, for example the length of the capillary is such that you have only one cell for such a length. During the filtration I think the haematocrit in the pore really does not bear a direct relationship to that haematocrit, because we do not have the length in the filter.

P.G. No further questions or comments? All right then we will move on to the next video presentation by Jean-Francois Stoltz.

JF.S. The Erythrometer is a commercial filtration system, which utilises the constant flow of an erythrocyte suspension with measurement of the filtration pressure as described by Leblond and Coulombe, with computer analysis and printout of data. Filters (Nuclepore or metal) are inserted into the filter holder and the system is primed with buffer. Buffer can flow either through the filter, or to an outlet for removal of air bubbles, by use of stop-cocks. The syringe pump is normally set at 5 ml/minute, and filtration pressure recorded graphically (maximum pressure 76 mm Hg). Four stages are involved. The patient's name, haematocrit and other basic data are entered into the computer. The system is set up and checked. Buffer is then filtered and the pressure (Pi) recorded. The red cell suspension in buffer is then filtered and the final pressure (Pf) recorded. The computer then prints out the relative resistance result,

$$R = \frac{Pf}{Pi}$$

The system detects the increased resistance of rigid red cells, e.g. in haemolytic anaemias or following fixation by glutaraldehyde.

A videotape of the method used by J-F. Stoltz followed.

P.L. How much does it cost?

JF.S. I think the actual price is around 25,000 francs. It is less in dollars, about 3,000.

H.S-S. What are the actual pressures you tend to reach, with for example a diabetic patient?

JF.S. The pressure I think is between 20 to 40 cm of water. The shear stress in the pores is between 500 to 5000 dynes /cm ^{2}. It is possible to modify the flow rate.

H.M. The volumetric flow rate was 5 cm^3 per minute?

JF.S. It is variable flow rate if you want.

H.M. I know, but the normal one that you use is 5 cm^3 per minute? (Yes).

J.S. The instrument clearly has the flexibility to use either 3 micron or 5 micron pore diameter filters, as distinct from Professor Hanss' haemorheometer which will function only with 5 micron filters because there is not a positive pressure above the filter. So it does give a certain degree of flexibility.

M.H. But you can apply a vacuum under the membrane, so you use what you like. But then you have high shear stress with 3 micron membranes.

H.S.-S. I think the two constant flow systems that we have seen (Marcel and Stolz), while of course hydrodynamically identical to the constant pressure system, run the danger of increasing the pressure when a blood sample is pathological. I think the great advantage of the constant pressure system is that this danger is avoided.

P.G. There do not seem to be any further comments or questions, and we can therefore proceed to the last video which is Paul Teitel's.

P.T. The 'Filtrometer' constructed by Mussler and Myrenne is a four-channel system designed to take up measurement data on flow rates. It incorporates a new type of U-shaped sample holder (patent applied for) in which the flow occurs upwards through the filter under a continuously decreasing pressure differential. Any kind of filter membrane can be utilized with this equipment. In each channel 250 substantive values for the fluid level are taken up by a photoelectric device. Data are stored in a RAM memory and then processed by a microcomputer according to different algorithms.

A videotape of the method used by P. Teitel followed.

M.H. I have two questions to ask you. First, what is the haematocrit range which you can measure? And secondly, how do you define the starting time of the filtration and when do you measure the initial rate, as regards to starting time?

P.T. I made here a combination of descriptions of both hardware and software. The first of your questions – this instrument has been designed to be used with any value of haematocrit. If we introduce a suspension haematocrit of 8% as in the case of Nuclepore sieves, we store in memory the 250 values which are measured in 8 minutes. We calculate the very first slope resulting from the first 5 points between 95% and 100%, which corresponds to the flow of pure buffer, and then we take another slope which corresponds to 90% of the whole range (in our case the whole range is a 30 mm water column) and this second slope (90%) is related to the first slope (95%) and out of this comes a printout of the result. As I mentioned before, we have residual information, which for the time being is not used. The instrument is versatile and takes up a great amount of information. What you do thereafter with all the information remains to be seen.

M.H. How do you know that the filtration is starting?

P.T. We continuously monitor the level, and the results of the reading as it is scanned at time intervals are displayed by digital display.

M.H. What is the suspension volume which you need to have a first initial rate measurement?

P.T. Approximately 27 microlitres of suspension.

H.S-S. We also have published *in vivo* tests of blood rheology, and we have had the good fortune to get a controlled stiffening of red cells by cross-linking spectrin with diamide. With these cells, which can be infused into animals or used in an isolated mesentery preparation as developed originally by Peter, we can show two things. When we infuse these cells into an animal, and then reduce the blood pressure to 35 mm of mercury (in other words, the animal is in shock), so the index of resistance goes up by a factor of 1.8. Then in the reinfusion period we have a hyperaemic response and so we have only a slight increase in resistance. Now when we stiffen the cells with diamide, we see little change in resistance until we reduce the pressure, when we have a very high resistance ratio, and in the reinfusion period we have no hyperaemic response at all – as a matter of fact we have great trouble in getting these cells to move! Now this was expected, because from all our *in vitro* studies we knew that as we reduce the shear stresses the differences between normal and abnormal cells become more pronounced. And from this we derived a philosophy which is incorporated in the machine. We have a simple rheological programme for the clinician, which is always set with the cheapest and the most reproducible force available, namely gravity, which is automatically controlled, gets us a large amount of potential information, and in which we are going through a range of low shear rates, and we are not increasing shear rates during the experiment thereby getting, for example, unplugging of the filters.

S.C. I would like to ask a general question to all the presenters this morning, as to whether you re-use the filters after each test of a cell suspension.

S.F. I discard after one use.

I.J. It is possible to re-use two or three times, but I prefer to change.

P.G. If you re-use them, how do you clean them?

M.H. We re-use them and we have never seen any difference between old and new membranes. We have done some controls on the membrane to see if the filtration conductance changes or not. The appearance of the filter changes slightly when we wash them many times. We wash them with diluted sulphochromic acid and rinse them thoroughly with distilled water, and then we dry them on a filter paper, and that is it. Usually we use them about 5 times on average.

J.D. Does anybody use plasma as suspending medium, and if so have they found that the second time round with the same filter you get a difference in the flow rate? Same filter, two filtrations of plasma, the second time you get a lower flow rate? With any system?

P.G. Can you give an answer to your own question?

J.D. Yes. In about 20% of cases if you pass the same plasma through the same filter you get a decreased flow rate. Don't ask me why!

M.H. We have tried from the beginning to use plasma as a suspending medium and in our first efforts we have succeeded in making measurements and the figures were always roughly the same as with buffer. But it is always very difficult to get good plasma samples, because you have all the protein aggregates inside, and so we felt that we had to pre-filter the plasma samples before using it as a suspending medium, but then we found that it was very difficult to filter plasma. Either you use very large pores and you are not very sure of what you are doing or else you use small pores (by small pores I mean one micron pore diameter Millipore filters) then it is very hard to push the syringe. It is a very complicated method and I do not know if it is worth it.

J.D. The phenomenon I described was in plasma after pre-filtration, I forgot to say that. Pre-filter through one micron diameter pores, and even after filtration in some patients you do get a variable flow rate.

J.S. When we take new Nuclepore polycarbonate filters, I suppose like most people we find that we need to discard one in 10 because when you filter your buffer through it you get a flow rate outside your usual range of acceptability. After we have used a filter and cleaned it with sulphochromic acid using Professor Hanss' technique, then we find that we need to throw out perhaps one in five.

I.J. A question about the role of plugging in two kinds of filtration methods. Do you think the use of gluteraldehyde-fixed red cells is a useful method to show the role of plugging? Here we have the results with several concentrations of red cells fixed with gluteraldehyde (Fig. 5.1). With Hanss' technique, we find that the sensitivity was about 0.02% fixed red cells/normal cells. The change was significant at about 0.04% fixed red cells/normal red cells. With the Kenny/Stuart technique the sensitivity was the same. So do you think we can interpret these results as that the two methods have the same sensitivity to plugging? If you look at the number of cells by pore, you have the same ratio with these two techniques. So do you think that we can say that these techniques are both sensitive to plugging, and if yes, do you think perhaps they are sensitive to white cell plugging?

P.L. I think that plugging by hardened red cells and plugging by white cells in the kinds of suspensions we use are not quite the same thing. I suspect that plugging with hardened cells will occur much more quickly. Despite the efforts in Professor Hanss' technique to avoid plugging by white cells (that is, measuring the very first few seconds of filtration so that you will avoid plugging by white cells maybe because they are in smaller numbers), you will probably get plugging with hardened red cells if you have any significant proportion of them in the red cell suspension. So I am not sure it is exactly the same thing we are talking about.

J.S. Dr Juhan's question, as she knows, is unanswerable, because there are two variables in the slide that she shows. These are the plugging effect by leukocytes, and the plugging effect of gluteraldehyde-fixed red cells. What she needs to do to be convinced by her own data is to repeat the experiment using white cell-free filtrates with both systems, and she will then be able to have a direct comparison of the sensitivity of the two techniques to a subpopulation of gluteraldehyde-fixed cells.

Sensitivity of methods to gluteraldehyde fixed red cells (Dr I. Juhan)

	% fixed RBC/ normal RBC	Fixed RBC/l	$\frac{IF}{m}$	p	Fixed RBC/ pore	WBC pore	RBC/ pore	$\frac{WBC}{RBC}$
Dormandy	0	0	0.357	—				
PCV 0.4	0.0001	5×10^6	0.348	NS				
Vol. 1 ml	0.0005	2.5×10^7	0.315	NS				
	0.001	5×10^7	0.271	<0.025	0.1	2	10000	1/5000
	0.005	25×10^7	0.111	<0.001				
	0.01	50×10^7	0.048	<0.001				
Kenny and	0	0	2.72	—				
Stuart	0.001	1×10^6	2.86	NS				
PCV 0.01	0.005	5×10^6	3.03	NS				
Vol. 18 ml	0.01	1×10^7	3.07	NS				
	0.02	2×10^7	3.18	NS				
	0.03	3×10^7	3.65	NS				
	0.04	4×10^7	4.12	<0.025	2	1	5000	1/5000
	0.05	5×10^7	4.62	<0.01				
	0.1	10×10^7	7.39	<0.001				
Hanss	0		12.29	—				
PCV 0.08	0.0001	8×10^5	11.62	NS				
Vol. 40 μl	0.001	8×10^6	11.35	NS				
	0.005	4×10^7	12.66	NS				
	0.01	8×10^7	12.53	NS				
	0.02	16×10^7	13.23	NS				
	0.03	24×10^7	14.16	NS				
	0.04	32×10^7	15.58	<0.01	0.03	0.015	75	1/5000
	0.05	40×10^7	16.48	<0.01				
	0.1	80×10^7	21.78	<0.001				
	0.5	400×10^7	59.30	<0.001				

Fig. 5.1

P.T. A short comment. We are now systematically using in parallel two types of filters in the instrument I have described: Nuclepore filters (as most people do), and large pore filters. And we have also made experiments concerning the identity of results which can be obtained with the two types of membranes. We have also done experiments in which we deliberately introduced gluteraldehyde fixed cells in our suspensions. It turned out that the sensitivity of the Nuclepore filters to a small percent of fixed cells, approximately 0.5%, was enough to clog the filter relatively rapidly – within a couple of seconds we had an arrest of flow. In the large pore tubes we observed for the first time irregularities in the flow pattern, that is to say a non-homogenous flow pattern, starting at 5 percent contaminating rigid red cells. I suppose, although I do not have evidence available, that leukocytes will also result in such flow irregularities in large pore filters.

M.H. I would like to make a point clear. I never said that my method was insensitive to membrane clogging. I said, and it is also in the abstract of the paper I have given, that the method is by and large insensitive to filter plugging, but there is a difference if you have say 5% of the cells which are stiff, which clog the membrane. In that case the initial rate would be decreased by 5%, roughly. So it is sensitive to plugging, but by an amount of 5% as opposed to large volume filtration, in which case the clogging goes on and then you have a very complicated situation.

H.M. Maybe the question I am going to ask is inappropriate. Last year I raised the issue of Nuclepore filters versus other types, and Paul has just hinted that there is a difference. I would like again to bring up the question; since Nuclepore representatives are not here, we can feel a bit more relaxed! The evolution of filtration has gone to Nuclepore filters. I think everyone in the room perhaps has used them, except perhaps Paul, and I have no commercial interest in any company but I am wondering if we should re-evaluate the use of Nuclepore filters as the only ones that are employed? Given that they look pretty under the scanning electron microscope; given that we can do analysis of flow through straight pores in a more reasonable fashion; it is however not obvious to me that it is the only filter material which will provide us with good answers. I think we have dropped the question, and I would like to have it brought up again. Is this the time to do comparative studies, or shall we postpone it until another time?

P.G. This was the topic of session 4 (types of filters) and in fact it turned out that the organiser of that particular session did not have any response from the group, except for his own, so it is exactly as you describe, the tendency to use Nuclepore filters continues!

H.M. Historically, we know that Shu Chien published early papers with Gregersen, and we all became very excited to see these holes that did not look like woven mesh, and then everyone else can do the analyses.

S.F. Why is Nuclepore not in our group? As last year.

J.D. We invited him and asked whether he would like to come (he was here last time, you remember), and he did not show any interest in coming. We could not kidnap him, we tried!

P.G. Thank you very much. I think now it is time for Dick Skalak to present his ideas on the analysis of results of filtration experiments.

R.S. Various indices have been proposed to express the experimental results for a variety of filtration test procedures for the filtration of blood cell suspensions. Insofar as such test procedures and indices are reproducible and show a variation with changes in properties of the suspension, these indices are equally valid in an abstract sense. However some indices may be more useful or indicative of the cell properties directly and may allow comparison between different physical test equipment and testing procedures. It will be preferable to have a dimensionless index rather than one with particular dimensions. It would also seem advantageous to have an index which is independent of the particular concentration of cells to indicate the intrinsic resistance added due to the presence of the cells individually rather than due to their numbers.

In such cases for which there is not any progressive plugging or partial blockage of pores, the filterability index proposed by Professor Hanss (1982) is probably the most useful expression to incorporate the aims mentioned above. In the usual Nuclepore filter test with progressive plugging, the equations and discussions below should be applicable to the first one or two seconds of the test during which extensive plugging has not yet occurred. The filterability index proposed by Professor Hanss may be written

$$r^F = \left(\frac{R_s^F}{R_0^F} - 1\right)\frac{1}{H_f} \tag{1}$$

where

R	=	resistance
F	=	values for the whole filter
H_f	=	feeding suspension hematocrit
s	=	values for the suspension
o	=	values for suspending fluid only

The index given by equation (1) is analogous to the intrinsic viscosity index, which is used in polymer chemistry to describe the influence of high molecular weight macromolecules on the viscosity of a suspension. In this case the intrinsic viscosity η_i is defined by

$$\eta_i = \left(\frac{\eta_s}{\eta_0} - 1\right)\frac{1}{c} \tag{2}$$

where c is the concentration of the polymer as a volume fraction, η_0 is the viscosity of the suspending fluid, and η_s is the viscosity of the suspension containing the polymer at concentration c. It can be seen that equation (2) is exactly analogous to equation (1), considering that the viscosity of a suspension is a resistance to shear flow analogous to the resistance of the suspension to flow through a filter.

In a recent paper by Skalak and colleagues (1982) the flow through a Nuclepore filter has been analyzed in more detail, indicating that when the feed hematocrit H_f is small, only a fraction α of the pores will contain a blood cell, and the remaining fraction $(1 - \alpha)$ will contain only suspending fluid. The analysis is based on the fact that the presence of the cell in a pore is evidenced by an increased resistance by a factor β over that for the flow of the suspending fluid alone. It can be shown from the equations given by Skalak et al. (1982) that the index given by equation (1) based on the entire filter is in fact exactly equal to a similar index based on the flow in a single pore only

$$r^P = \left(\frac{R_s^P}{R_0^P} - 1\right)\frac{1}{H_P} \tag{3}$$

where P indicates values for a pore and H_P is the hematocrit in the pore containing the cell, i.e.

$$H_P = V_c/V_P \tag{4}$$

where V_c is the volume of one blood cell, and V_P is the volume of one pore. It is remarkable that the indices given by equations (1) and (3) can be shown to be exactly equal using the equation given in Skalak et al. (1982) in the case where there is no plugging of the pores. This indicates more directly that the index suggested in equation (1) is indicative of the properties of a single blood cell flowing in a single pore. It is further remarkable that the experimental data indicate that the index given by equation (1) is relatively independent of hematocrit up to hematocrits of at least 8% (Hanss, 1982). In high polymer solutions the divergence from a constant intrinsic viscosity occurs at much lower concentrations.

The relative resistance ratios used in equations (1) and (3) may be expressed in terms of a variety of experimental results. As indicated in the working group report on red cell deformability of 1981 the following relative resistance expressions are all equal.

$$R^F_{REL} = \frac{R_s^F}{R_0^F} = \left(\frac{p_s^F}{p_0^F}\right)_{Q=\mathrm{Const}} = \left(\frac{Q_0^F}{Q_s^F}\right)_{p=\mathrm{Const}} = \left(\frac{t_s^F}{t_0^F}\right)_{p=\mathrm{Const}} = \left(\frac{V_0^F}{V_s^F}\right)_{p=\mathrm{Const}} \tag{5}$$

where the subscript p = constant or Q = constant refer to tests in which either the pressure or flow rate is held constant during the test. The superscript F is used again to indicate a test involving measured values for the entire filter. The times t_s^F, t_0^F are measured times of flow for a fixed volume at constant pressure. The volumes V_0^F, V_s^F are volumes passed in a filter for a set fixed time. The use of the relative resistance as expressed in equation (5) allows comparison of many different kinds of tests.

Similarly in the case of a single pore the relative resistance of a pore containing cell to that of the same flow in a pore containing only suspending fluid may be expressed in the following form

$$R^P_{REL} = \rho = \frac{R_s^P}{R_0^P} = \left[\frac{p_s^P}{p_0^P}\right]_{Q=\mathrm{Const}} = \left[\frac{Q_0^P}{Q_s^P}\right]_{p=\mathrm{Const}} = \left[\frac{t_s^P}{t_0^P}\right]_{\substack{p=\mathrm{Const}\\ V=\mathrm{Const}}} = \left[\frac{V_0^P}{V_s^P}\right]_{\substack{p=\mathrm{Const}\\ t=\mathrm{Const}}} \tag{6}$$

In equation (6), ρ is the individual single cell pore resistance ratio defined by

Skalak *et al.* (1982).

Another point of interest which allows comparison of different tests follows from the equality of equations (1) and (3). This is a relation between transit times observed for the filter as a whole or for a single pore. The relation is

$$\frac{t_s^F}{t_0^F} = [\frac{t_s^P}{t_0^P} - 1]\frac{1}{H_P} + 1 \qquad (7)$$

The superscripts and subscripts in equation (7) have the meanings as used previously. The times t_s^F, t_0^F are times required to pass a given volume of suspension and suspending fluid respectively, as measured, for example, in the Hanss apparatus (1982). The times t_s^P, t_0^P are the times required for the passage of a single cell through a single pore and of a particle of suspending fluid (based on mean velocity of fluid flowing in a pore without a cell) such as has been reported by Keisewetter and colleagues (1982). If the conditions of the two tests are comparable in avoiding plugging and in the flow rates used, the equation (7) should be very closely fulfilled.

It is emphasized that the above discussion and equations should allow comparison of a variety of tests on condition that the tests are performed in a range in which there is no appreciable plugging of pores during the test period. In the case where plugging is present a more elaborate theoretical analysis is required (Skalak *et al.*, 1982). In such cases the indices indicated by equations (1) and (3) above may not be the most relevant or appropriate for the situation. Probably other indices should be derived for the situation in which there is appreciable pore plugging.

H.M. I think Dick's analysis is really clear, and what astounds me (and Shu indicated it earlier) is that this is not true for any sort of polymer system, that is the independence of the RF or the intrinsic viscosity or the specific viscosity values with concentration. You always see deviation from linearity, and that is the reason, as Dr Hanss pointed out, you need to extrapolate to zero concentration and zero shear rate. And I am wondering is this true all the time, or is it only true for normal cells under certain conditions? What are the limits? I mean certainly Dick's analysis with the straight line says that this is true, and you can vary beta and get different values, but for a given beta or for a spectrum of beta's it is always true. When does it fail in pathologic situations or whatever?

S.C. I think Holger is probably going to comment on the pathological situations, but I would like to give a general answer to your comment, Herb. I think in the polymer solution viscometry we do it in three-dimensional space, and it is a volumetric measurement. And here I think the thing that simplifies it is the geometric constraint. The cell has to go in in a certain way so that you do not have this complication with three-dimensional volume effect. And that is why you are able to keep it in almost the same situation up to a fairly high concentration, unless you change the geometry when you have two cells in the same pore as Dick indicated.

H.M. Let us change the geometry slightly, let us make the pores thicker and longer and more tortuous. OK, what do we expect there?

R.S. I am very optimistic. I think you are going to find that any of these methods, and any shape of filter within some reasonable pressure range (meaning well below haemolysis, and high enough to prevent aggregation) that you are going to find this index can be gotten out of any old filter.

H.M. I know that the index can be gotten out, that is easy. The question is the independence of particular concentration, up to what seems to me 20% by volume.

R.S. When I saw that this index can be gotten out, I mean that you will find a single index over a range of concentrations which will be at least up to 10%, and perhaps as high as 20% was surprised.

H.M. So the implication then is that up to 20% haematocrit the haematocrit level is only determined by your ability to measure pressures easily, or timing easily, and you need not worry if it is 4, 8, 10, or 12?

R.S. Also by the kind of plotting where you plot it first against haematocrit and just look at the data. Shu is going to show more like that again, I think, this afternoon. You showed it yesterday. That way you can check yourself very quickly experimentally how a particular filter pressure range either agrees or does not agree with this straight line dependence on haematocrit.

H.S-S. I think one of the other reasons why we have this surprising insensitivity to haematocrit is the fact that we have virtually no interaction between cells up to that high concentration, except possibly if we are talking about an abnormal entrance behaviour. And so the only comment I would like to make (and this is based on thorough experimental evidence) is that as we go down in pressures and at the same time avoid aggregation we are seeing more difficulties of the cells to enter. We therefore have to insert one important caveat: all of this applies only under the condition where the approach, entry, passage and leaving of the cell is uninhibited. And there is good evidence that disease is characterised by disturbances of these. Now there are very important practical implications. Because most of the patients we are looking at have a spleen, and the spleen somehow seems to be engineered to remove rigid cells, and since the cells we take from a patient's vein have within the last 15 minutes once passed the spleen, the cells we are looking at appear to be selected in the spleen for the very property we are trying to establish. Therefore it is not surprising that, with the exception of severe haemolytic anaemias and burned patients and a few other exotic diseases, we do not see grossly rigid cells. We are trying, especially in diabetes and other metabolic diseases, to detect subtle changes, and it is very important of course that we really can compare the resistances as a function of the applied shear stress. Because we are talking about highly non-Newtonian systems, and therefore we have to understand that there is an enormous discrepancy in the literature because people have not checked for the adequate hydrodynamic conditions. In other words we have to keep in mind that a cell which is only mildly affected, and that seems to be the case in diabetes, must necessarily evade detection by a majority of the apparatuses used, whereas others (which employ lower shear stresses) are likely to uncover this, simply because we are dealing with these highly shear-stress-dependent-behaviour cells.

M.H. I wanted to comment on the polymer viscosity. Indeed it is the deviation from the straight line at a few percent for normal proteins. So what is the difference with the red blood cell? First, I am not quite sure that it is haematocrit-independent up to 20%: we have not done the measurement. Maybe it should be done, but between 0 and 8% it is linear. There is a problem. What is the difference? The difference is that when you use a protein, the volume of the protein is considered as an excluded volume, around which the solvent has to flow, and the viscosity increment is a measure of this additional drag around the molecule. On the contrary for red blood cells the red blood cell is not a rigid particle, so it is quite normal that it is different from the protein molecule. I think that red blood cells should look like droplets, nearly as free as water, and indeed we calculated some very rough approximation transit time of the cells through the pore with our measuring system, and we found a transit time which was the same as Kiesewetter's technique extrapolated at the same pressure, and this transit time is of the same order of magnitude as the transit time for the solvent. So there is not as much difference between the mechanical properties of red blood cells and solvent, as there is in the case of protein and the solvent. And then I would like to add a little additional comment on the minus 1, which seems to be a trivial reduction when the ratio is high. When you have got a filtration ratio which is, say, 100, then you have got a bad measurement. Because the measurement must be so that the ratio is near 1, otherwise it means that you get all the complicating factors coming along.

S.C. As Dick pointed out we should use the relative resistance. I think in the early reporting of the results, people usually used either the flow of the suspension and the transit time, the flow time, or the pressure. More recently people are normalising, dividing by the suspending medium to obtain relative resistance. But what Dick said is that even that will not give you the intrinsic property of the cells. What *will* give you this is what he said: taking the relative resistance minus 1 and then correcting it for the pore haematocrit. Pore haematocrit is the haematocrit divided by the ratio of the cell volume to the pore volume. Then you end up with an intrinsic property. That is the intrinsic property of the cell during this particular filtration test. It is still dependent on the filter. But at least you normalise it for the cell concentration and for the suspending medium. Now these two parameters are linearly related. The relative resistance is linearly related to this intrinsic parameter, but the linearity varies with the haematocrit. For example when you use 1% haematocrit this dependence is much stronger than at 20%, which is obvious because the haematocrit goes in the denominator.

Now the question is how do you test it? If you test it with 1% haematocrit, you get a very low relative resistance reading. If you test it with 20% haematocrit, you get a very high relative resistance reading. So if you just record relative resistance it would not help. But if you correct for the haematocrit then it gives back an intrinsic property. Then the question is, what haematocrit should you use? This came up several times, and this is dictated by the sensitivity of the instrument. If you have a very sensitive instrument that can measure very small relative resistance, you can go to a low haematocrit, like Dr Hanss is using, and then he gets a magnification effect. Any error, or any sensitivity, is magnified. You magnify the error, you magnify the sensitivity, so here is the compromise. How sensitive do you want a method to be, and how good are your methods? So you have to compromise in choosing the haematocrit. So if the reading is not very accurate we had better use a haematocrit such as 10%. In our *pressure* measurement, we favour something like 10% because we feel that is where we can get accurate measurement of the pressure. So the choice of haematocrit is really linked to what Dick has said about the intrinsic parameter.

G.L. Well, I feel that I have drawn the short straw in trying to summarise the mass of information which we have had this morning! For a start, I do not propose to summarise the elegant analysis which Dick Skalak has just given us. It is all clear in our minds (I think) and so I will opt out of that and go straight to the presentations. We started with Sandro Forconi who showed us beautiful pictures and music and chianti. He is using of course the original Reid/Dormandy method and he stressed as he did yesterday the importance of temperature. There is a surprising lack of correlation in his hands with the white cell count, and perhaps other investigators should just check this, using his technique of minimal storage and keeping the sample at 37° C, because it is very surprising.

We then had Professor Hanss' machine demonstrated. I think we are all now aware of the principle of Hanss' method, where there is very rapid measurement of the initial flow rate in a constant pressure system. From the data so far according to Hanss, it seems that there is no definite relationship of this measurement to the white cell count. There was however some discussion as to whether his machine is still sensitive to pore clogging, and I think this remains an open question until we have more work. Laboratories using this technique will note that the majority of this group would appear to accept any of their papers submitted for publication. They will, however, notice who they should send their manuscript to. And I am sure Tony will pass on that information to them. As Ehrly mentioned, widespread use is no reason for any method to be the correct one, and it has been said that he who is right is a majority of one. And that is a general comment.

Going on to Tony Marcel, he gave us his usual elegant presentation, cautioning against the apparent simplicity in the use of constant flow methods. He is obviously having problems with the method, in which however he is still using plasma as a suspension medium. I think from this meeting the complexities of analysis of pressure tracings are apparent, and we have to consider exactly what to do with the constant flow systems and the pressure tracings. This leads us on to Professor Stoltz's machine, and in contrast with Professor Hanss' machine this is now measuring pressure at constant flow. So that after the very first pressure measurement, we are again on to pore clogging. It looks a nice machine, now apparently available commercially for $ 3000, or equivalent, and I am sure we all look forward to hearing about the general experience with the first standard or automated constant flow method.

We then had Paul Teitel. Paul's approach, as is now well known, is a microcomputer-processed measurement of flow curves, using a decreasing pressure head system and monitoring the level of suspension. Initially he has been using his large bore filters, which again he took us through in his first presentation this morning, but the system also appears capable of using Nuclepore filters. The system has shown interesting results in terms of homogeneity of flow in the large bore filters, and the fluctuations with decreasing pressure which are picked up by this sophisticated, but now readily available, form of analysis with microcomputers. Certain cells in this system appear to behave like granules of sand flowing intermittently as in the hourglass timer.

So in summary there are now a variety of systems available for distribution or use among several centres, and this is a development which I think we would welcome, because we are all aware of very conflicting results in the past five years as regards so-called 'filterability' of red cells in various clinical conditions and after exposure to various drugs. These conflicting results, it is now clear, can be due to several differences between centres, but some of them relate to hydrodynamic conditions in filter systems and the timing of measurement. It is apparent from all yesterday's discussions that you must try to consider two things: the true red cell deformability which you may pick up at the start of whatever system you use, and secondly plugging, particularly with white cells, which you are on to thereafter. I see that the major advantage of these standard machines is to allow better comparison between laboratories, and what I look forward to in the future is to reading studies of clinical conditions in which there is maximal interest, namely diabetes and different kinds of vascular disease and their risk factors, and perhaps to be able to make a better comparison of results from different laboratories which might now start to incorporate (not necessarily use absolutely) such standard equipment as we have heard about. Because other factors being equal, one might be more certain then that when you read different results from different centres, these might be due to perhaps different populations of patients rather than to differences in the filtration procedures. But having said that, these machines do clearly measure very different things, and we must keep clearly in mind what exactly is measured in each system. And equally important are yesterday's discussions on the sample preparation. Paul uses computers, and in the computer world there is the saying which goes 'rubbish in rubbish out', and we have to keep in mind what exactly we are putting into these elegant machines with their sophisticated analysis. And finally it has been most interesting to compare our presenters' use of videos, and I am sure that we should give them a brief round of applause for their time and trouble spent in making them.

Report from the Groupe de Travail sur la Filtration Erythrocytaire (French Filtration Group)

P.G. I think we should start and enter into Session 6 which is really Tony Marcel's report from the French Filtration Group (FFG).

G.A.M. Thank you, Mr Chairman. As I suppose we all know, there is a FFG and we meet more or less every year and in June we had our 7th meeting. There will be a book published of the 7th meeting with summaries in English. There are about 110 members of the FFG now and it all started after the publications on the Reid and Dormandy apparatus as we set up apparatuses of these types all over France in the university hospitals so that clinicians with an interest in the field could appreciate the results. I am not going to give, of course, a pure summary of the communications given at the 7th meeting. I am going to tell you what I felt when the communications were made, which is of course extremely biased and artificial but hopefully sincere. Professor Hanss with his young co-worker Koutsouris gave a very interesting communication on the physico-chemical factors influencing red cell filterability. I think all of you should know that there are already three Theses which have been published on his method, which I suppose are not in most bookcases but have a lot of very valuable information. Those really working in this field should perhaps read these. The Hanss index is the time of passage of cells minus time of buffer on time of buffer corrected for haematocrit. Figure 6.1 shows the influence of osmolality, pH, temperature on cells and on ghosts and, what I have thought was very original, the influence of pCO_2. There were some discussions on the influence of Tris buffer and phosphate buffer on results but as far as I have read this is one of the only papers on influence of pCO_2 on red cell deformability and therefore should not be neglected. Another very interesting point was the comparable results with ghosts and whole cells on the filterability index. At the meeting Jean-Francois Stoltz presented his new apparatus which was there for demonstration. The group of Quemada showed data on influence of morphology of red cells in bank blood on relative viscosity at both high and low shear rate. They also presented their recent data on abnormal aspects of thixotropy and viscoelasticity in patients with scleroderma, which has not been published to my knowledge. Hurez published correlations between filtration time and plasma proteins: C

Influence on red cell filterability (as measured with the Hanss Hemorheometer) of osmolarity and pH.

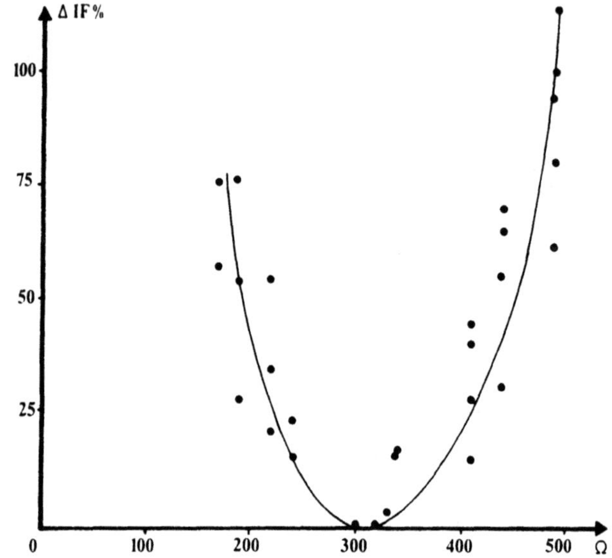

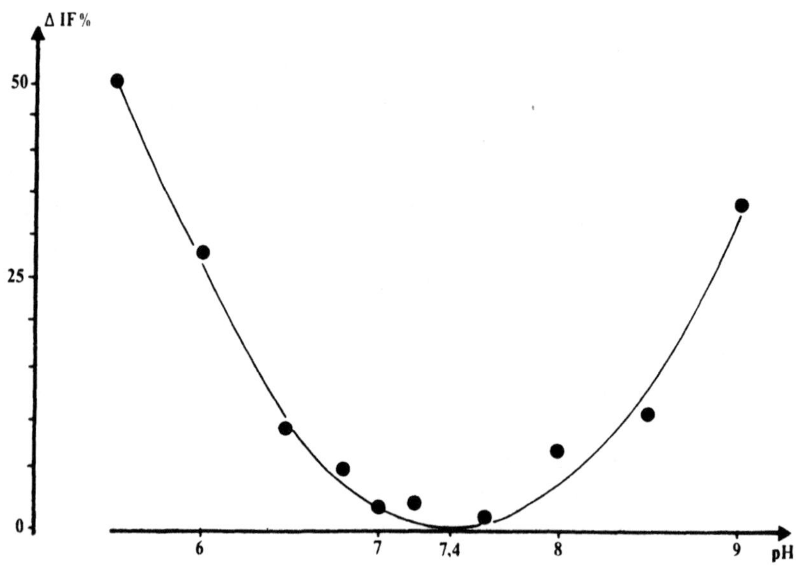

Fig. 6.1

reactive protein and orosomucoid. It has been pointed out many times that whole blood filtration correlated with acute phase reactants such as fibrinogen, Von Willebrand's factor (as Boisseau has shown), CRP or orosomucoid in this more recent paper. Droulle communicated on red cell filterability and haemodialysis patients using washed resuspended red cells and showed correction by haemodialysis of decreased filterability and of abnormal electrophoretic mobility. There was a long discussion on the influence of ionised calcium on these facts and correction of ionised calcium by haemodialysis. Those are the more fundamental communications. Then we came to clinical communications. What was original in this meeting is that up to now we had always been wondering whether the anomalies found in peripheral arterial disease were linked to other things than red cells or linked to diabetes and so it was interesting to have two communications, one from Juhan and the other from Delaunay showing that patients with peripheral arterial disease without diabetes and studied with the Hanss method could have reduced filterability or red cell deformability, use the word you want. I think we agreed (cf. p. 151) that publications using the Hanss method could be accepted if the word deformability was used. The conclusions of I. Juhan were that patients with peripheral arterial disease have a reduction of deformability whatever technique is used (Fig. 6.2). What was very agreeable was that not only the classical methods of filtration with non-washed red cells or with washed red cells showed significant decreases of filterability or deformability in patients with peripheral arterial disease but also the Hanss method showed significant decreases of deformability in patients with peripheral arterial disease. We tested the Hanss method in seven different centres in France and normal people usually have a Hanss index around between 9 and 10, here the mean was 13.73 in these patients with peripheral arterial disease without diabetes. Delaunay also checked the Hanss index in patients with peripheral arterial disease and without diabetes. He showed as Irene Juhan had that there were disorders in this index in these patients and he tried to correlate these with phosphorylation of membrane proteins by running SDA page tests and interestingly showed that there was absolutely no correlation. Le Devehat looked at whole blood filterability as a prognostic index in diabetic macroangiopathy and he showed the prognostic value of whole blood filterability (Fig. 6.3). The group of Deshayes in Orleans studied the evolution of whole blood filterability and clinical severity index one year after stroke. And they found the best prognostic index associated with the least filtration reduction. This is interesting because it also goes with what Boisseau had published two years ago measuring whole blood filtration on patients with stroke. He realised that those who had the worst figures of filtration two or three days after their stoke were those who were most likely to die within two weeks. So again the test had a clinical value although it didn't have a clearcut biological significance. As a sideline, but not without interest there have been quite a few publications on the various iodine

The time filtration index (I.F.) for the Hanss hemorheometer is increased in peripheral arterial disease, indicating reduced red cell deformability.

$$I.F. = \frac{Tsusp. - Tbuf.}{Tbuf.} \times \frac{100}{Ht\%}$$

Author	Normals	n	PAD	n	p
Juhan	11.76±0.80	11	13.73±3.39	20	= 0.037
Delaunay	9.9 ±2.4	10	14.7 ±4.7	10	<0.01

Fig. 6.2

related contrast substances used in arteriographs. One of these substances, hexabrix, was investigated and in 38 patients showed no change in platelets, fibrinogen, thromboeleastograph, plasminogen, antiplasmin and whole blood filtration was checked before and after in 38 patients and was not changed at all by this substance which may make people feel a bit more safe than certain other substances. Then we have some communications on pharmacology. Boisseau studied fixation of fibrinogen on human red cells and showed inhibition by

Evolution of blood filterability in diabetic macroangiopathy (from Le Devehat).

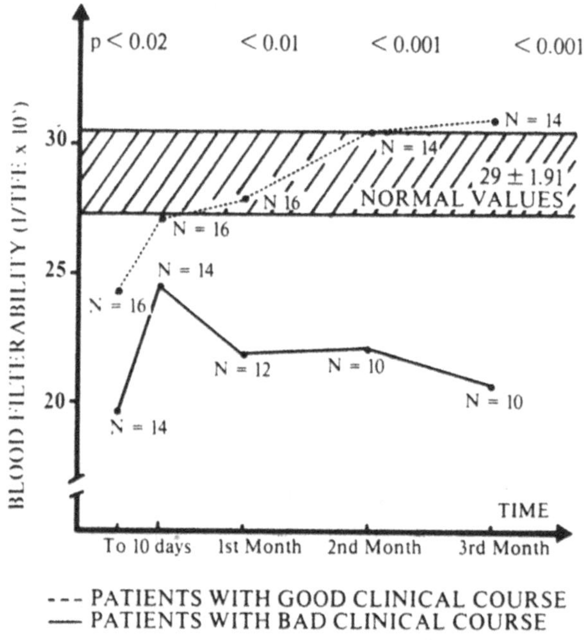

Fig. 6.3

supra-pharmacological doses of pentoxyfiline. Pentoxyfiline at very high concentrations induces up to a 40% decrease of the fixation of fibrinogen on to red cells. But this again is not at pharmacological levels. The group of Schmid-Schonbein represented by Seifge reporting on the work with Kiesewetter and Schneider reported on the effects of pentoxyfiline on measures in single pore erythrocyte rigidometer *in vitro*, *in vivo* and in disease states. Pentoxyfiline will give 24.7 msec medium passage for a control at 37.6. What's interesting is the low concentration here of pentoxyfiline used which corresponds to 10^{-6} M. Up to now we have never been able to demonstrate *in vitro* activity of pentoxyfiline at concentrations below 10^{-4} M, which shows that with this method you can demonstrate activity of a drug at 10^{-6} M *in vitro* which for us was very interesting. Another very exciting point for the people interested in pentoxyfiline is that theophylline had no action. *In vivo* patients who have received the drug and who have quite evidently before therapy reduced medium passage time corrected during therapy and relapsed after the discontinuation of therapy with still a certain residual effect. Another exciting thing was medium passage time in various states: stroke seems to reduce considerably the medium passage time; diabetes and multiple sclerosis also. In liver diseases the group of Hanss showed correlation of his index and certain membrane lipids. Gueguen and Driss showed correlation with whole blood filterability to be positive with membrane non-saturated fatty acid concentration but negative with saturated fatty acids in patients with cirrhosis (Fig. 6.4).

P.G. Thank you very much Tony. Anybody want to add a comment?

J.D. I was interested in Dr Juhan's finding of decreased filterability in claudicants who were not diabetic. Now what happened if you added insulin as you have described that adding insulin does make the red cells more normal in diabetics, does it have any effect on non-diabetic claudicants?

I.J. I don't know but it could be bad for their arteries!

J.D. Yes. I wasn't advocating it as a treatment of arterial disease.

J.S. You will remember that yesterday I passed around a paper that is in press in *Clinical Haemorheology* showing that PVD patients have normal deformability by our technique. You can understand it's a little difficult for me sitting where I am this afternoon to put up an opposing view but there is an essential difference between the two studies in that we studied vascular disease outpatients in the steady state and our controls were normal people who are obviously out of hospital. Dr Juhan's patients with vascular disease were in hospital and her controls were taken from age matched people who are also in hospital. So the populations in the two studies are not comparable and that may well explain the difference.

J.D. Even less comparable are your two techniques for measuring red cell filterability.

J.S. Agreed.

In patients with severe chronic alcoholism there is a positive correlation between red cell membrane concentration in unsaturated fatty acids and whole blood filterability, and a negative correlation for saturated fatty acids (from Gueguen and Driss).

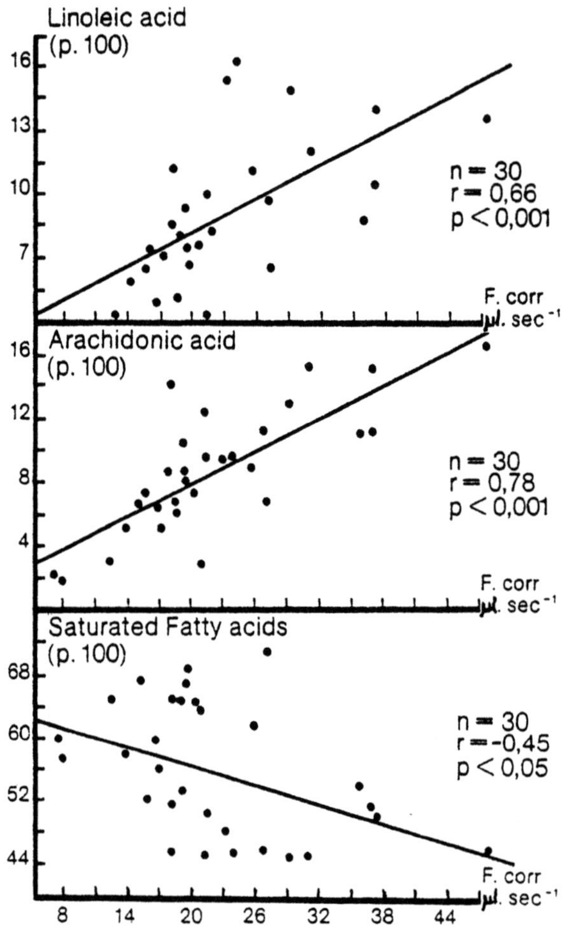

Fig. 6.4

P.G. Further questions? Albrecht Ehrly.

A.E. In 1976 we studied patients with chronic vascular disease with our technique which is almost the same as the one we use today. The surprise was that patients having macronagiopathy and diabetes had the same filtration rates as patients without diabetes. Has anyone had experience in the meantime which could underline or oppose our findings?

P.G. We will come back to the question of diabetes in the following session.

S.F. I think it is not very difficult to explain the difference in red cell filterability when we study different populations because in our experience, and I will show it in my presentation this evening, red cell filterability can rapidly change in patients and is clearly dependent on the stage of the disease.

P.G. We will come back to some of these aspects in discussing the clinical significance of filtration tests, which is the next session, and John Dormandy will start by defining, I hope, the criteria of clinical relevance and doing that in five minutes is a marvelous task.

SESSION 7

Clinical relevance of filtration tests

J.D. We have so far discussed some of the variables in filtration techniques reproduced in this diagram. We have tried to assess the relative importance and contribution of these different factors and how we can interpret the results produced by combinations of these factors. In this session we want to apply ourselves to the question: are the results, irrespective of the exact technique of filtration used, clinically relevant? I mean by that, are the results of any filtration test useful in the prediction, management, determining the prognosis of the disease or the development of new forms of therapy? What we have in the filtration test is a kind of black box into which we pour the blood and out of which comes a number. You can approach such a phenomenon in two ways; so far we have been approaching it from the basic science point of view – what is actually being measured inside that box? But we can also look at the number we get out of the box and see whether it is clinically relevant. I would suggest that these two paths should be followed simultaneously rather than consecutively. They are interrelated and if we can acurately define the clinical states which produce abnormal results new light may be thrown on what we are actually measuring, and vice versa. I suggest that in the following presentations dealing with specific diseases we should consider the evidence under these five headings, which I believe are the criteria of clinical relevance:

1. Is an abnormal RCF a risk factor possibly related to the development of the disease?
2. Is it part of the pathological process which characterises the disease?
3. Is it an indication of the severity or the incidence of complications?
4. Does it relate to prognosis?
   and finally, perhaps most importantly
5. Does it help in the development of new forms of treatment?

P.G. Thank you. The next presentation will be by John Stuart on the possible clinical relevance of red cell filterability in sickle cell disease.

J.S. There have been a large number of elegant studies on *ex vivo* samples from patients with sickle cell disease in the steady state which have given a lot of basic information about the haemorheological abnormality of sickle cell patients. The problems arose when investigators tried to move on from this stage to actually studying patients during a vaso-occlusive crisis. Figure 7.3 shows the theoretical change in any acute-phase reactant during the 7 to 14 days after the onset of a sickle cell crisis (but it could equally well be surgery or an acute infection). The vertical axis represents the percentage change in any acute phase reactant such as the plasma fibrinogen level or the leucocyte or platelet count. The slide also shows that although the temporarily raised level of such a reactant returns to the normal range in many patients at the end of the first or second week, in some it remains raised, and it is our particular thesis, in Birmingham, that patients with chronic vascular disease not only have an acute phase response but they also have a chronic phase response. A patient with peripheral vascular disease with a steady-state elevation of plasma fibrinogen, gets an additional rise during the acute phase of a thrombotic event and then goes back to a steady state, but that steady state is still above normal. You might think that that does not apply to sickle cell disease but remember that patients with homozygous sickle cell disease have lost their spleens because of autoinfarction. Therefore a patient in the steady state of sickle cell disease will continue to show a slightly raised platelet count because he has no spleen.

Robert Hebbel from Minneapolis has shown that sickle cells adhere to cultured endothelial cells during the acute crisis period. But this may be the con-

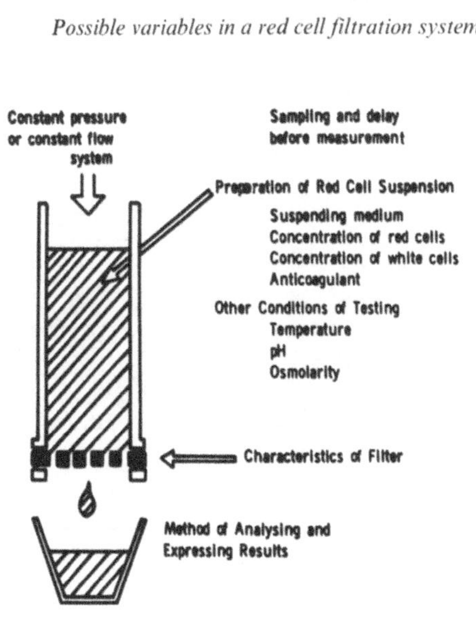

Fig. 7.1

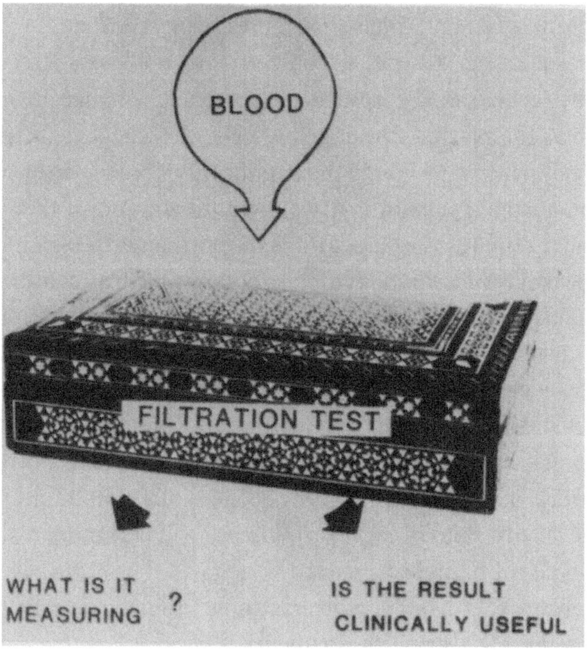
BLOOD
FILTRATION TEST
WHAT IS IT MEASURING ?
IS THE RESULT CLINICALLY USEFUL

Fig. 7.2

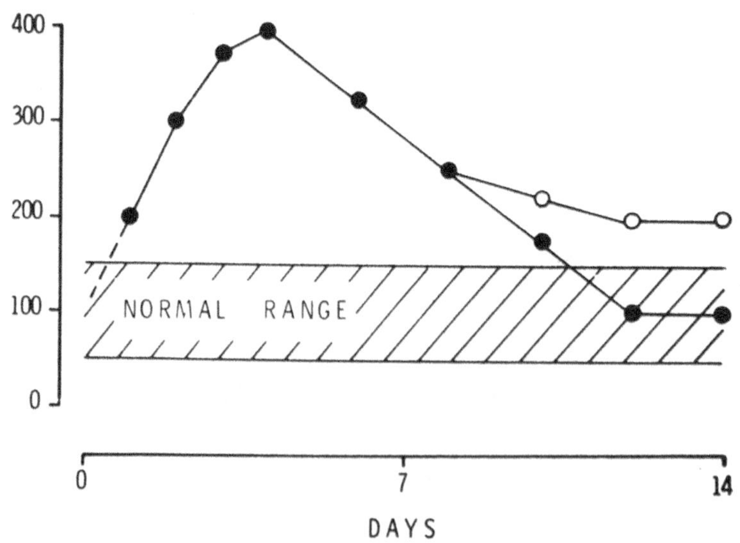
400
300
200
100
0
NORMAL RANGE
0
7
14
DAYS

Fig. 7.3

sequence of the acute-phase rise in plasma fibrogen level. So, whatever type of red cell metabolic study you carry out, you must take into account the acute phase response.

The next slide (Fig. 7.4) shows the mean values for 10 sickle cell crises followed serially from days one to nine, as well as the values in the same patients during the steady state. If you look at the whole blood viscosity (at the relatively high shear rate of 128 reciprocal seconds) there was no significant change compared with the steady state, until one week after the beginning of crisis. In contrast, the red cell filtration ratio using the Birmingham technique of washed red cells was already significantly elevated on day one. Now everyone here will say, after this morning's discussions, that this could be a white cell effect. In fact, the white cell count on day one was not significantly different from the steady state, although by day two it was significantly raised. Clearly somebody should repeat the study using a washed red cell suspension that is free from contaminating leucocytes.

The next slide (Fig. 7.5) shows that this type of study is clinically relevant in that we were lucky enough to study one patient before a crisis. These are the pressure curves for his washed red cells in phosphate buffered saline. 'a' is the patient's pressure curve when he was in the steady state, 'b' shows the increase in the pressure 24 hours before a painful crisis and curve 'c' is the pressure recorded during the third day of his crisis. A similar result was reported by Dr Rieber in BLOOD in 1977. His patient had a prolonged filtration time, using 3 micron pore size filters, two days before the crisis and the filtration time became even worse during the actual crisis. So to look at washed red cells and to filter them in parallel with the development of sickle cell crisis is obviously important.

The other study that we have done is to look at these patients in the steady state and to look at the interaction between another inherited disease and sickle cell disease. Some patients inherit alpha thalassaemia as well as homozygous sickle

Sickle cell crisis		Crisis						
	Steady state (19)	Day 1 (6)	Day 2 (10)	Day 3 (10)	Day 4 (10)	Day 5 (10)	Day 6–7 (10)	Day 8–9 (10)
Whole-blood viscosity mPas ($128\ s^{-1}$)	5.80 ±0.34	5.90 ±0.47	6.00 0.67	5.80 ±0.43	5.96 ±0.50	6.09 ±0.53	6.20* ±0.58	6.23* ±0.72
RCF ratio	6.15 ±1.48	8.21* ±2.77	8.37** 2.39	7.61* ±2.12	7.89* ±1.97	8.43** ±2.55	7.33* ±1.41	6.80 ±1.21

* $p<0.05$; ** $p<0.01$

Fig. 7.4

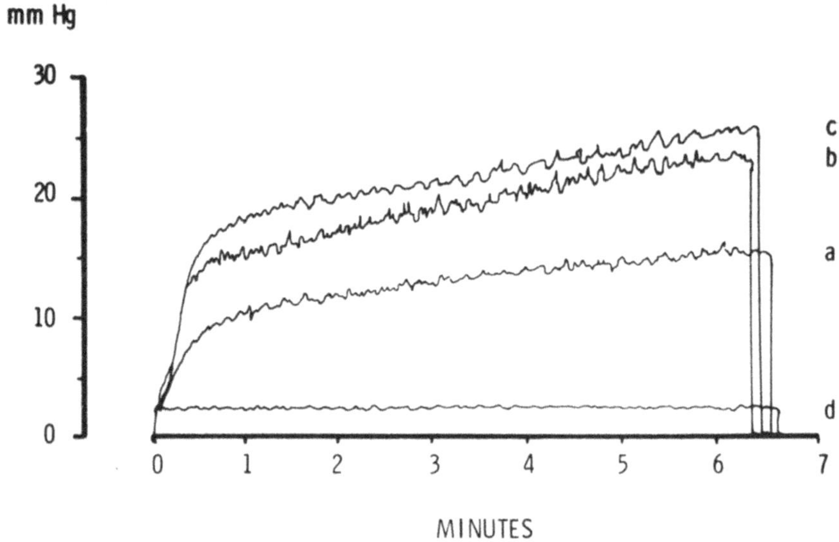

Fig. 7.5

cell disease and if you have the two diseases together then the alpha thalassaemia decreases the production of globin chains. These sicklers will have red cells with less haemoglobin, lower MCV, lower MCH and lower MCHC, and the patients may be clinically less severe. This was reported by Higgs this year in the *New England Journal of Medicine*. Because of that study we carried out the following investigations in conjunction with Graham Serjeant at the MRC Laboratories in Jamaica and with Professor Weatherall's Nuffield Department of Medicine in Oxford.

We found that the sickle cell patients with thalassaemia had significantly better filtration, the cells passing through 5 μm pores more readily than the patients without thalassaemia. There are several explanations for this: the patients with thalassaemia and sickle cell disease had smaller red cells with less haemoglobin per cell and fewer reticulocytes, so these cells should filter more easily and this may explain the reduction in clinical complications such as leg ulcers and the acute chest syndrome.

P.G. Tony Marcel has the first question.

G.A.M. There was no fetal haemoglobin in the alpha thalassaemics at all then?

J.S. The mean fetal haemoglobin levels in these patients was less than in homozygous sicklers with a normal alpha globin gene compliment. That was shown by Higgs in the earlier study.

G.L. John, while you are doing your next study of looking at a white cell free system in a sickle cell crisis, would it be possible to use the logarithmic correlation you described yesterday, where you plot the log of the white cell count against your filtration index, and apply that retrospectively to your data in this study or would that not be valid?

J.S. You cannot use the same regression line because yesterday's regression line was calculated using normal red cells. You would have to take a regression line from the sicklers and honestly I do not think it is worth it. It would be better to get rid of the white cells altogether.

P.L. You told us that you had calculated a final pressure resistance and an early pressure resistance from your pressure curves. If there is any influence of white blood cells you could have seen it in the difference between those two. Did you in fact see a difference?

J.S. No, but our initial pressure is not measured as early as the initial pressure from the Columbia University team presented yesterday. They talk about an initial pressure in the first second or two, our initial pressure is measured much later.

S.C. All our pressure analyses presented yesterday were done on normal blood, I mean normal AA, cells and their beta value, rigidity value is quite different from the white cell. Here the question is how rigid are these sickle cells? If they are close to the white cells we may not be able to see any separation between the two. They may mix in together. If they are sufficiently different you can resolve them by graphic analysis; I think that is the problem. One question that I have is were these oxygenated sickle cells?

J.S. That is right. We bubbled oxygen into them so that the blood was well aerated and pink. That is different from the Rieber study from New York in which he progressively deoxygenated the cells. We have tried to get rid of the effects of deoxygenation on sickle cells.

J.D. I am intrigued by the patient you measured before his crisis. At that stage, when his filtration was already abnormal, was he clinically totally asymptomatic? Secondly, were any other measurements carried out at that time abnormal?

J.S. Like I suppose you mean the white cell count?

J.D. Yes, and fibrinogen.

J.S. We did not look at them. The patient rang up the next day in pain and obviously he had been in an asymptomatic pre-crisis stage when we had studied him the day before.

P.G. We will now have another haematologist's view of the clinical relevance of red cell filterability by Paul Teitel.

P.T. Some 20 years ago the first clinicians to be interested in what is now termed deformability were haematologists; they tried to explain the splenic sequestration of abnormal red cells (and hence their accelerated removal from the circulation) by a rheological mechanism. A relatively great number of early publications have indeed shown that in many different haemolytic disorders red cell filterability is abnormal. In publications made in 1964 and 1967 I have tested the clinical validity of filterability measurements (in large pore filter systems, i.e. polymicroviscometry) by comparing them with data derived from *in vivo* studies on the life span of Cr^{51}-labelled red cells. Although not directly warranting the conclusion of a cause-to-effect relationship, the statistical analysis of this data disclosed existence of significant correlations. I must confess that in view of these earlier findings I felt rather uneasy when I saw the many recent reports on diminished red cell 'deformability' in the most different pathological conditions. If abnormal red cell deformability is primarily understood as a common denominator of haemolytic disorders, this would implicitly mean that in all circulatory discorders associated with abnormal filterability there should also be a haemolytic component. Moreover, it would also mean that the main indication of drugs said to improve red cell deformability would be treatment of haemolytic disorders. I am suggesting that in circulatory disorders associated with an abnormal filterability we should also take a look at the possible existence of such a haemolytic component: this could either be perfectly compensated by a moderate increase in the erythropoietic function of the bone marrow, or actually be absent following from a certain degree of splenic insufficiency (circulatory exclusion). Comparing different methods to assess the 'deformability' of red cells, it is increasingly apparent that different methods and filters are seeing different rheological features; we are also becoming aware of the fact that data obtained with a particular method cannot be equated with data obtained with another one. To correctly assess the rheological behaviour of abnormal red cells, we should probably utilize simultaneously several methods in order to find out which factor is decisive in which pathological conditions.

Assuming now that a normal spleen removes rigid red cells from the circulation, we will also have to accept the notion that we will find in the periphery only a cell population highly selected with respect to rheological behaviour. In other words, if the spleen is normal there will be only a small likelihood to find gross rheological abnormalities in blood samples obtained from vascular provinces in which the circulation is normal. For many years now to investigate minor red cell abnormalities in haemolytic disorders, haematologists have been first submitting them *in vitro* to abnormal biochemical conditions such as incubation (i.e. metabolic depletion in the autohaemolysis test) or oxidative stress (incubation with acetylphenylhydrazine). By the same token we hold it necessary to assess also rheological abnormalities after 'stressing' the red cells in different ways. As a matter of fact, we have found great inter-individual differences in what could be called rheological response (or reactivity) in such 'stress models' simulating conditions thought to occur in vascular provinces with a deranged circulation. We are therefore suggesting to utilize this approach both for clinical diagnosis and pharmacological studies.

P.G. Herb Meiselman.

H.M. I would like to offer just a couple of quick comments. Because of my creeping age and the greyness of my beard I decided to look at some of the questions of age separation of cells relevant to Dr Teitel's work on survival time and the question of what determines cell survival time. I think what this may lead to perhaps is that for some populations of cells in certain patients we might want to do more than measure either whole blood or washed cell filtration but also look at different fractions of the cells from the patients. All the geometric data which we obtained on young and old normal erythrocytes show no differences between young and old erythrocytes. The surface area goes down with age, but so does the volume and the surface to volume ratio does not change. The smallest pore through which they can traverse does not change with age, it is identical between young and old normal cells. What does change are some of the mechanical behaviours of the cell membrane measured using micropipette techniques or a flow channel technique. The shear modulus of the membrane, that is its resistance to stretch at a constant area, was the same in unfractionated cells, young or old cells measured either by the micropipette or by the flow channel. So in terms of the membrane's ability to stretch at constant area there is no difference between young and old cells. But if you ask how quickly can the cell respond to a deforming force, that is its viscoelastic time constant, it turns out that there is a fairly substantial and highly significant difference between young and old human erythrocytes. The time constant for shape recovery for the older cells is much longer than that of the younger cells. You can go on to calculate a membrane surface viscosity which is about 50–60% higher in the older cells than the younger cells. This suggests that survival of cells may not be entirely a geometric factor but may be a membrane mechanical factor such as the rate of their response to mechanical forces.

Now the other thing we became interested in was the fetal red cell, that is cells taken right from the cord, which as you know have a 60 day survival time. The next slide (Fig. 7.6) shows the results obtained from the top and bottom fractions for either normal adult cells or for fetal cells, top meaning the young cells, bottom being the old. The dashed lines are the neonates and the solid lines are the adults. The unlabelled points in the middle represent the unfractionated samples. Interestingly, deformation measured in a cone-on-plate rheoscope was the same in unfractionated neonatal and unfractionated adult cells. But the younger Neonatal cell are more deformable and the older neonatal cells are less deformable in the comparable fraction from the adult individuals, I guess what I am suggesting from all of this is whether we should look not only at an unfractionated sample but begin to look at density or age fractionated samples as well?

P.L. Just one question to Paul Teitel, which I also raised, you may remember, last year at this meeting. How can we find so many disease states in which using one method or other there seems to be a decreased red cell 'deformability' and yet

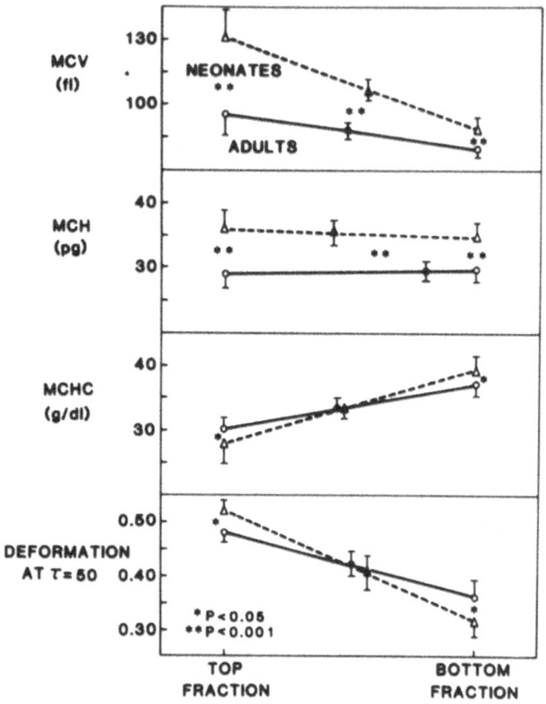

Fig. 7.6

not have any evidence of splenic red cell destruction in these individuals? I think one of the possible problems is that as we all know there are serious limitations as to how precisely you can detect small changes in red cell life span *in vivo* using the radio chromium labelling techniques. I would suggest perhaps another approach to this would be to use some enzymatic method to evaluate mean red cell age in the population of cells and see if it correlates with red cell filtration or deformability. This could be an interesting study for example in diabetics or people with peripheral vascular disease. We could then see whether the spleen really acts as a nice little filtration device *in vivo*, the same way as we want to interpret these results *in vitro*.

S.F. A question to all those present. Has anyone experience with subjects without a spleen?

P.L. Yes, we have made a certain number of measurements on splenectomised individuals and although there is some variation the average value that we get with our technique was slightly higher in terms of resistance than with normal cells. But it is not a large difference.

A.B. There is one study showing diminished red cell survival in diabetics which fits in with your comment.

J.D. To answer Professor Forconi's question. There was one study that I know of in renal failure where the red cell filterability was decreased slightly but when you removed the spleen it fell tremendously, something like 80% change in filterability after splenectomy in the same patient.

M.H. I have a question to Holger related to multiple sclerosis. There is some data showing that in the single pore technique the transit times are elevated in multiple sclerosis and I wanted to know your point of view about the influence of the electrostatic field coming from the membrane charge density on the single pore or any filtration technique. Because investigators are showing that the red cell charge density is lower in multiple sclerosis. So my question is whether the transit time is related to the surface surface interaction between the filter membrane and the red blood cell membrane?

H.S-S. We are toying with this idea and trying to find a good experiment. We have the gut feeling no, but we have no definite proof.

G.A.M. There are many papers describing an abnormal distribution of plasma fatty acids and plasma phospholipids in multiple sclerosis, so you could easily imagine that there is an exchange with red cell membrane lipids.

P.G. Let us now return to clinical relevance, and Gordon Lowe's presentation.

G.L. This is a two part presentation of which this is the first part. Lots of patients come into hospital for general surgery. About a third of these develop deep vein thrombosis if you scan them by the conventional radioactive iodine labelled fibrinogen test. We looked at various clinical factors and many laboratory tests, including whole blood filtration by the original Reid-Dormandy method, prior to surgery in 63 patients. There was no difference between patients who subsequently developed deep vein thrombosis and the two-thirds of patients who did not develop deep vein thrombosis. So from the point of view of prediction, this simple robust test did not seem to be of any predictive value; neither was blood viscosity, haematocrit or a whole variety of laboratory tests. We were able in the same paper to show that age and obesity were quite a good index for predicting deep vein thrombosis. Now, I do not know why we become old and I do not know why we become fat, and I suspect nobody does. But whatever the basis for age and obesity they have a good predictive value, and I would make the point that you do not necessarily have to know everything about the mechanism of an effect whether it is a clinical measurement or laboratory measurement, for it to be useful.

Turning to diabetes, I described yesterday our technique where at the time when we take the initial pressure reading we have shear stresses of about 17 pascals. We used the index P_i over P_b, where the initial cell pressure is corrected for variation in filters by dividing by the buffer pressure. Diabetic patients were studied at six week intervals for 18 weeks. The first thing we wanted to see was whether there was a difference between human insulin and animal insulin in terms of their effect on red cell deformability. This may have been relevant because human insulin has been shown to bind differently to red cells compared to porcine insulin. In fact we found no difference at all in this short-term study between diabetics on human insulin and diabetics on animal insulin. So we then lumped all the data together and looked at the relationship between recent diabetic control, as measured by the percentage of glycosylated haemoglobin and deformability and we have found a relationship to control. Of the 22 insulin dependent diabetics studied, 20 had no detectable diabetic complications. The 22 controls were matched for age, sex, smoking and John Stuart will be happy to know that there was no significant difference in their white cell counts. The diabetics did have higher haematocrits and plasma viscosities but of course these are corrected for in the filtration system used. The diabetics had significantly more rigid cells than the control group at all times. And a difference emerges if you look at control. Now we looked at this in two ways. Firstly we did a comparison within each diabetic subject looking at the RCF when the glycosylated haemoglobin was at its highest, a mean of 11%, and at its lowest, a mean of 9.5%. You can see that this spontaneous fluctuation over the 18 week period in recent diabetic control does appear to be associated with decreased red cell deformability because you get apparently more rigid cells when the glycosylated haemoglobin is at its highest compared to when it is at its lowest (Fig. 7.7).

H.M. You are saying that if the patient is well controlled then you see no difference between their filtration and that of control donors? So that if one wanted to see differences in diabetics, the maximum difference would be in the poorly controlled individuals.

G.L. That is correct. As I say, where we took all the patients at each patient's highest glycosylated haemoglobin compared to each patients' lowest glycosylated haemoglobin. Now there is another way you can look at the effect of

Red cell filterability (P_i/P_b, where P_i = initial pressure of cell suspension and P_b = buffer pressure) in 22 diabetics during a randomised study of animal and biosynthetic human insulin, compared to 22 non-diabetic controls. NS = not significant.

	P_i/P_b	
Non-diabetic controls	1.15±SEM 0.05	p<0.01
Diabetics – baseline	1.35±0.04	
– after 6 weeks animals insulin	1.33±0.07	N.S.
– after 6 weeks human insulin	1.33±0.10	
– highest glycosylated haemoglobin (mean 11.0%)	1.50±0.08	p<0.02
– lowest glycosylated haemoglobin (mean 9.5%)	1.23±0.06	

(Study performed in collaboration with Drs J.M. Leiper, A.C. MacCuish and W.G. Manderson, Diabetic Unit, Glasgow Royal Infirmary.)

Fig. 7.7

control by comparing patients who were generally poorly controlled to patients who were well controlled. And again we find a similar relationship. So on this data from uncomplicated insulin dependent diabetics you can see that there does appear to be a relationship of the initial pressure in this constant flow system to recent control as shown by glycosylated haemoglobin. This relationship is not seen if you measure the pressure later at say six minutes, because pore clogging in diabetics and normal appears then to be similar. I think there are two messages: you have to look at diabetics early to see differences in filterability and this may explain some of the discrepancies in the literature about whether or not filtration is abnormal. The other source of confusion in previous studies may be that red cell filterability depends on the degree of control. If you study well controlled diabetics you may not see any difference but if you study poorly controlled diabetics then in our experience you do appear to see a difference. Thank you.

P.G. Now let us turn to Adrian Barnes' account of diabetes.

A.B. I was asked to do three things: firstly to give you a potted history of deformability and diabetes, secondly to consider the fact whether measurement of deformability may be relevant in predicting clinical outcome and thirdly I am asked to shut up after 10 minutes, and I was asked to do them in that order. The first person to filter diabetic red cells would appear to have been Jørn Ditzel, who filtered whole blood through Millipore filters in 1970 and found the passage of whole blood to be slow. A few years later Holger Schmid-Schönbein and his colleague Dr Volger were the second group to report filtration studies in diabetics and suggested that badly controlled diabetics tend to have impaired filtration. Shortly afterwards, Albrecht Ehrly and John Dormandy and I reported rather similar findings in diabetic patients with complications. Since that time there have been an increasing number of studies on filtration and the 'take home' message from these studies appears to be that metabolic imbalance is associated with slow filterability of red cells under most test conditions. In addition, if patients have widespread complications filterability is also found to be impaired. An additional interesting finding from Irene Juhan is of course that insulin can affect filterability. Although the mechanism has not been fully elucidated, it is certainly accompanied by an increase in intracellular ADP. What is not quite clear is whether red cell filterability is still abnormal if you normalise metabolism and look at diabetics who have no vascular or microvascular complications. In this slide (Fig. 7.8) I compare results obtained with other techniques claiming to assess red cell deformability. Using Dintenfass' TK value we found that diabetic cells are just about the same as normal cells. Sirs' centrifugation technique suggested that all our diabetic red cells are far more flexible possibly due to the high levels of fibrinogen which influences his technique. Now, the micropipette method, here again we have some interesting controversy which I am sure Dr Meiselman will comment on. Don McMillan uses 4 micron micropipettes in which he oscillates red cells up and down along a horizontal distance

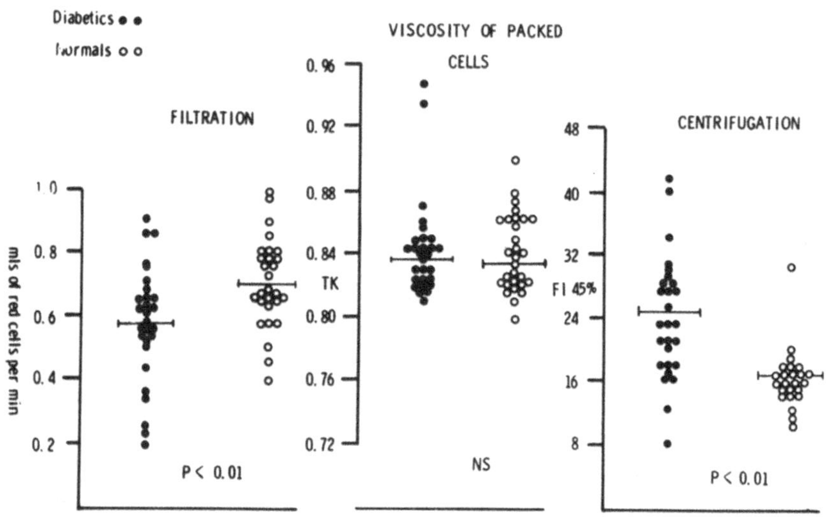

Fig. 7.8

of about 130 microns with a frequency of three seconds. He finds the pressure resistance to be 50% increased in diabetic patients. If he then blows the red cell out of the end of the micropipette and times the shape change to achieve a biconcave disc, he finds something like 70% delay in the red cell in diabetics. Dr Meiselman has tried to reproduce these data, Paul La Celle has tried to reproduce these data, and we have looked at this without finding any significant increase in diabetics. The discrepancy really remains to be explained.

The second question is: do the rheological abnormalities come before the complications and are they a good predictive factor? Now what we have done is that we have taken 15 diabetic patients and we have improved their metabolic control by strapping them to an infusion device which gives them continuous subcutaneous insulin and they can get extremely good metabolic control. These are all patients who had retinopathy and we have made serial retinal photographs so that we can analyse in detail capillary closure and all the other complications over a period of time. The study has only lasted eight months so far, and is not yet complete, but in summary we have been unable to implicate filtration tests as being useful in determining who is actually going to deteriorate. Before we all get carried away with the idea that rheological abnormalities are the cause of diabetic problems, I would just like to show this slide (Fig. 7.9) which shows the many different factors which have been put forward to account for deterioration in diabetic microcirculation. Obviously we have to consider rheology as part and parcel of the whole scenario.

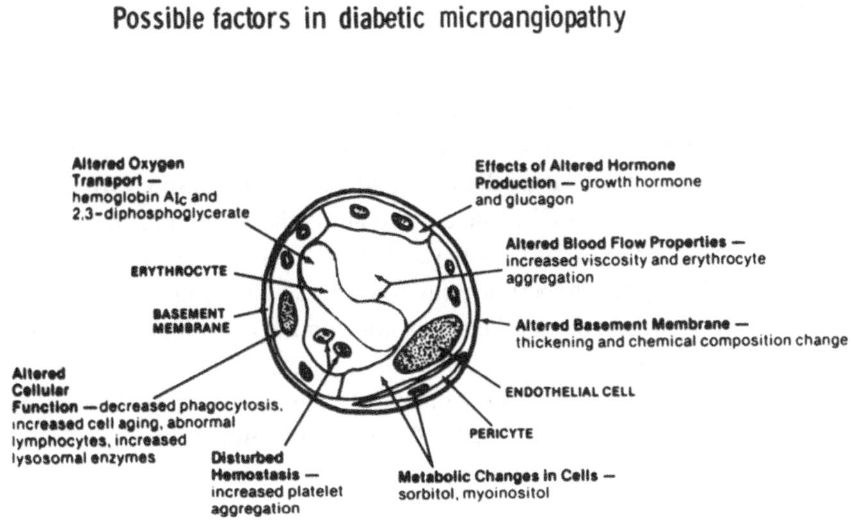

Fig. 7.9

M.H. I would like to show our results in a large scale study of diabetic patients in a general hospital in Bobigny. The population studied is over 300 patients but we only have 200 complete results so far. We have about 100 patients who are insulin dependent and 100 who are non insulin dependent. On heparin samples the average filtration index for diabetic patients is significantly different from the non-diabetics and there is a difference between the insulin dependent and the non insulin dependent diabetics. A curious result is that the filterability decreases when the patient's haematocrit increases although we do not know why. There may be a simple explanation, for the haematocrit may be measured with a kind of Coulter counter which is affected by the deformability of the cells. There was no correlation using EDTA samples, but this I have argued already yesterday. However, we have found no correlation with complications or with haemoglobin Alc, which is at variance with most results in the literature. Another unusual result is that there is no correlation with age or sex so that there may be no need to match for age or sex in filtration studies.

P.G. Thank you very much Dr. Hanss. The floor is open for discussion.

J.D. Obviously the information we still need is the kind of information presented by Adrian looking at the deformability or filtration and then following the patients clinically, not just for a few months but for several years. I would like to ask Dr Juhan or anybody else if they have looked at diabetics a year after measuring their red cell filtration and correlated filtration with the clinical progress?

I.J. No we have not.

M.H. We planned a one year study which will not be completed till the end of this year.

P.L. I know what you refer to when you say that deformability may influence measurement of MCV with Coulter counters. It would seem to me, although I do not have actual figures, that one would have to think of very large changes in red cell deformability, much larger than those which we can measure with filtration techniques to alter the MCV. The other point is that as you probably are all aware, in uncontrolled diabetics with very high plasma glucose levels the red cells are used to living in a hypertonic environment so that you can have falsely elevated MCVs when you put them in isoton and then in a Coulter counter.

S.F. In our experience if we look at patients in acidosis and the same patients after four months when they are controlled there may well be a correlation between haemoglobin Alc and red cell filterability. But if we take the same patient on the second day when the glycaemia may be well controlled, we may find that RCF is better but haemoglobin Alc is still the same and it is quite impossible to find a correlation between the two parameters. We think that there may be an impaired filtration during acidosis and in the acute state or when there is a major vascular complication but in the average well controlled diabetic there is no abnormality in the filtration.

A.B. Could I ask Shu Chien a question? One is obviously quite struck by what happens to white cells in Brånemark's study and of course the key pathophysiological event in diabetes is occlusion of capillaries in the retina because that precedes proliferative retinopathy. Therefore is it possible that abnormal white cells might participate in this and has he any data on white cell function in relation to high sugar levels, insulin and diabetics?

S.C. I do not have any.

G.A.M. I went through one of Brånemark's films with him and saw beautiful pictures of red cell adhesion to endothelium. So already before any publications on this subject he had the pictures.

H.M. My question is prefaced by two comments which I think we may all agree on. First of all that filtration measurements, by whatever technique, are exquisitely sensitive to surface to volume ratio of the cell; and secondly, I think we would all agree that the Coulter device is a very expensive machine full of artefacts which Coulter never tells you about. My question now is the one that Pierre has already raised and that is the volume of the erythrocyte when taken from a diabetic patient who is in poor control. I am not sure that the diabetic cell does not change its volume when resuspended in an artificial medium. It may swell less if the patient is in better control or if you have over a period of time dropped the glucose by insulin treatment so that the cell in the patient is in an almost normal glucose environment. Perhaps we ought to throw away the Coulter computer portion and do old fashioned MCVs with a cell count and haematocrit in the plasma or in the buffer you are using or both.

J.S. The other problem with the Coulter counter is that the amount of plasma trapping between normal red cells may be different when you have rigid cells.

P.L. How different do they have to be in order to change the Coulter measured MCV significantly?

J.S. Probably quite rigid.

H.M. But you know that for a manual cell measurement the trapping does not change from 200 milliosmoles to 800 milliosmoles. So I have got a computerised Coulter too, but it is nice to do the old fashioned method.

H.S-S. I think we should also recognise that Jørn Ditzel was the first to describe and try to quantify the red cell aggregation aspect of diabetes and this of course is what the clinician sees in retinopathy. Volger measured the relative flow rate of a 10% suspension of red cells in plasma and here (Fig. 7.10) you can see that the filterability is independent of complications such as nephropathy or inflammation. By contrast in the next slide (Fig. 7.11) the shear resistance of red cell aggregates is seen to be dramatically increased especially in those many patients who have an inflammatory disease and I think we are simply looking at an acute phase reaction. This slide (Fig. 7.12) shows the results obtained with our single erythrocyte rigidometer before and after filtering the blood as in the modified Reid-Dormandy technique. In the upper panels, before filtration, you

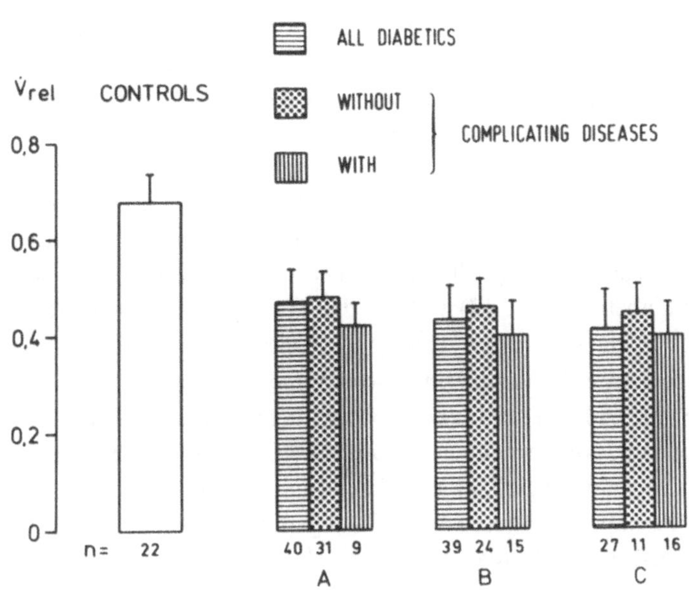

Fig. 7.10

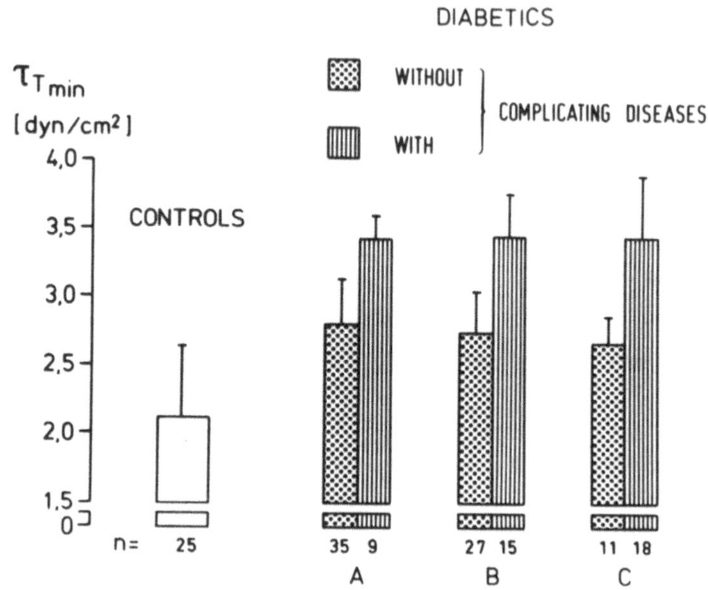

Fig. 7.11

see a small sub-population of slow cells in the right, and you can also see that the population of cells that go between 0 and 10 milliseconds is very low. Interestingly, if we now filter these cells as in the modified Reid-Dormandy technique, then the distribution is changed and we see more fast cells on the left between 0 and 10 and very few slow cells. In other words we are very sure that there are sub-populations of cells and I am afraid Herb that if I read your paper correctly you did experiments on only six cells per patient, sucking a little membrane into a micropipette, which is very much more complicated, and I do not accept that the so-called shear elastic modulus can be measured with this system. So in a recent study of diabetics (Fig. 7.13) we looked at many parameters and for example in the diabetics the yield stress is about five times higher than in the controls. We have of course an elevated plasma viscosity and a dramatic difference in the mean passage time. All you need is an appropriate technique to pick it up.

P.G. Thank you very much. I think Herb, I guess you will have to have a chance to defend yourself, at least defend the micropipette.

H.M. Perhaps the easiest way, without getting into a long discussion, is to tell you, Holger, that in the diabetic cells the shear modulus was not measured with a micropipette. It was measured with a flow channel technique.

H.S-S. It is the same thing. It is a question of bending and shearing.

H.M. No, it is absolutely different. Bending is not involved in the micropipette

Effect of red cell filtration (Reid-Dormandy) on distribution of RBC pore passage times

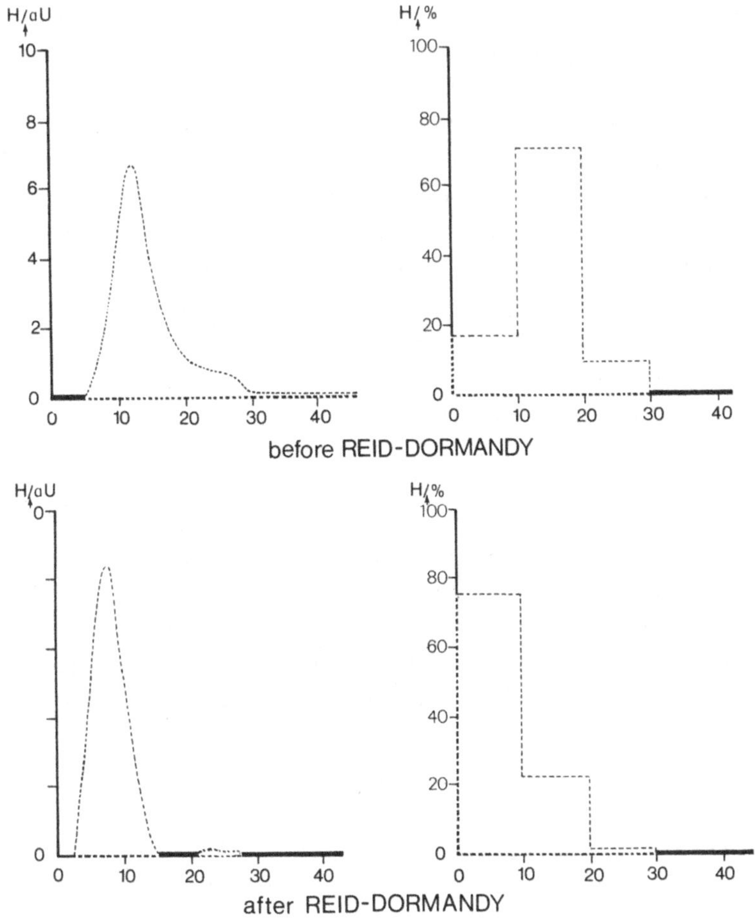

Fig. 7.12

	Control	Diabetics	
λ y (mPa)	1.1 ±0.5	5.3 ± 5.1	S4
α rel	3.46±0.42	4.60± 1.04	S1
λ Hkt (%)	45 ±4	45 ±6	S0
Pl (mPa s)	1.26±0.08	1.44± 0.14	S6
FA	16.8 ±3.8	31.8 ± 5.6	S7
Extent of red cell aggregation			
TM (ms)	24.9 ±7.3	55.6 ±13.4	S2
% occluding red blood cells	1.3 ±1.1	16.2 ±14.4	S7

Fig. 7.13

aspiration for shear modulus. In any case we used the flow channel for the diabetic studies.

S.C. Could I just speak to the micropipette issue. I am not trying to defend it but I think the micropipette technique is designed to test some specific aspects of the behaviour of the cell which is mainly the membrane shear elasticity and viscosity. These parameters may not change in a lot of situations, but the fact that they remain normal is not a reason for saying that that test is no good.

H.S-S. But it is no good for differentiating between diabetics and normals, which is what we are talking about.

S.C. All right, but you did not preface it with that sentence.

H.M. Excuse me, but hidden in the arguments for example of haemoglobin Alc is the possibility of some interaction between it and the membrane and the way to find that out is to measure membrane properties.

S.C. I think if you want to analyse the behaviour of the whole cell you have to assess whether the membrane is normal or abnormal. If it is normal you can then concentrate on the viscosity of the interior and the surface to volume ratio.

H.M. Exactly.

P.G. I hope you will allow me to steer the ship out of these dangerous waters and call on Peter Buchan to talk about neonatal jaundice.

P.B. I am going to tell you a nice simple straightforward story, which does fulfil some of the criteria for clinical relevance that John put forward. I think as I tell you the story you will see it is relevant to the first two criteria and certainly it has resulted in a change in our treatment not only in our hospital but I think generally throughout the country. One of the biggest problems that we face in obstetrics is the patients accusing us of interfering with them and causing harm when most doctors like to think they are doing good. We do in fact have fairly clear evidence that iatrogenic factors are responsible for the creation of neonatal jaundice. There have been a large number of studies done showing that the dose of oxytocin given and the duration over which this dose is given is associated with the extent and duration of the neonatal hyperbilirubinaemia. People have known about this association and many different theories have been put forward to try and explain why these babies have an increased level of jaundice. But none of the theories were confirmed. When doing general rheological studies in pregnant women I was looking at the altered rheology of labour and when I got out the statistics looking at what happened in spontaneous labour as opposed to what happened with oxcytocin induced labour, it immediately became apparent that there was a significant difference in the fetal erythrocyte deformability between the induced group and the spontaneous labour group. It appeared that oxcytocin, or something to do with the induction of labour, was reducing deformability in both fetal and maternal blood. So I undertook a fairly large study looking at various haematological and biochemical values in cord blood in three groups of patients: those with an elective caesarean section where the baby was being snatched unchanged from its mother's womb, spontaneous labour without the use of drugs and oxcytocin induced labour with no analgesic drugs other than pethedine. There was no difference in haematocrit, erythrocyte deformability by the Reid-Dormandy method using cells suspended in their own plasma, plasma bilirubin, plasma haptaglobulin level, lactic dehydrogenase and osmolality between elective caesarean section and spontaneous labour (Fig. 7.14). So it was clear there must be some critical difference due to oxcytocin induced labour. The haematocrit was significantly lower, plasma heptoglobin level was even lower than usual, the lactic hydrogenase was higher and the osmolality was lower. So there was clear evidence of a haemolytic process going on over a number of hours and these babies had all been exposed to oxcytocin for between eight and 14 hours. This increased haemolysis was associated with an erythrocyte deformability which was significantly lower. So now the conclusion that we felt like making from this was that the reduced erythrocyte deformability was in some way responsible for the reduction in haematocrit. Now how could this be? Well, I think the answer may lie in the osmolality because oxcytocin has an action very like vasopresin reducing the osmolality. You will notice that it is significantly lower in pregnancy, about 10 milliosmoles lower, than in the non-pregnant state; and in women who had oxcytocin induced labour it was lower still. So I went on to look *in vitro* to see if there was any immediate direct effect of oxcytocin on erythrocytes and the pharmacological dose of oxcytocin that we use in induction labour is round about 300 microunits per millitre, so I looked

Haematological and biochemical values in cord blood

Cord blood	Elective caesarian section Mean±SE (n)	Spontaneous labour Mean±SE (n)	Oxytocin induced labour Mean±SE (n)	p*
Haematocrit	0.52±0.012 (15)	0.53±0.013 (40)	0.47±0.014 (40)	<0.001
Erythrocyte Deformability Index ml/min	0.83±0.03 (15)	0.81±0.04 (40)	0.61±0.06 (40)	<0.001
Plasma bilirubin u mol/l	31±1.2 (15)	33±1.3 (40)	38±1.5 (40)	<0.001
Plasma haptoglobin g/l	—	0.091±0.024 (25)	0.023±0.006 (25)	<0.01
Plasma lactate dehydrogenase I U/l	—	223±8 (25)	346±25 (25)	<0.001
Plasma osmolality mosmol/l	286±4 (15)	290±6 (40)	277±6 (40)	<0.001

* p was derived using Students t-test comparing oxytocin induced with spontaneous labour

Fig. 7.14

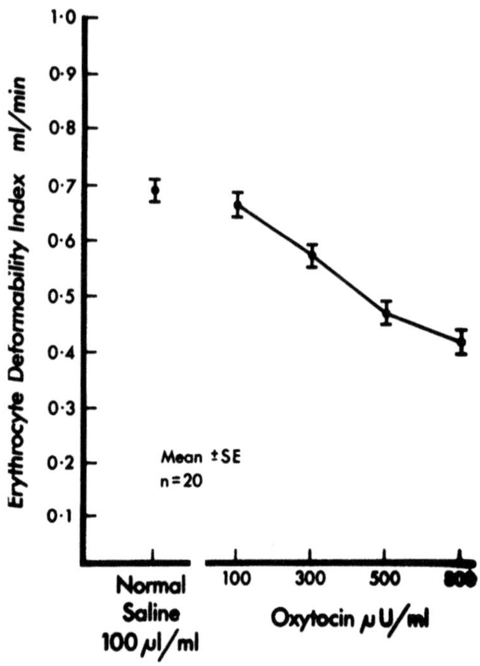

Fig. 7.15

above and below this range and we could see a dose related response, after incubation for two hours at pharmacological (Fig. 7.15). It seems probable to me that oxcytocin affects the fetal red cells by altering the electrolyte balance across the membrane secondary to an osmolar effect and hence leading to increased breakdown and jaundice. The implications of this from a clinical point of view are to reduce the dose and the duration of exposure to oxcytocin. We usually achieve this by combining oxcytocin with prostaglandin, which allows the total dose of oxcytocin to be reduced significantly. Obviously I had to check that prostaglandin did not itself have an adverse effect. So I did this *in vivo* with both prostaglandin and bipuvocaine because a lot of ladies having labour induced had an epidural; and *in vivo* I could show no difference in patients who were just having an epidural or patients who were just having prostaglandin for induction of abortion. *In vitro*, bupivocaine produces no change in erythrocyte deformability. Looking at prostaglandin E2, the physiological or even the pharmacological levels are in the range of picogrammes and I got no effect at all with those very low levels. But even at the much higher range shown here, I saw no consistent change really (Fig. 7.16).

And then on the time related incubation the normal controls showed the general fall-off that I saw with my method and with these initially I saw a fall in deformability with prostaglandin E2 and then after a short while the prostaglandin was perhaps metabolised within the red cells. So my conclusions from this were that oxcytocin is bad for babies, therefore it is reasonable to reduce the total dose of oxcytocin by giving the ladies a certain amount of prostaglandin, which has no effect on red cell deformability.

P.G. Thank you very much. Discussion.

S.F. Very interesting data. Neonatal jaundice is out of my field of interest but there seems to be a correlation between jaundice and carboxyhaemoglobin. Is there a relationship between carboxyhaemoglobin and filterability?

P.B. That has certainly been looked at in cigarette smokers. Cigarette smokers in many studies have been shown to have a reduced filterability. Equally, people have looked specifically at carboxyhaemoglobin levels, and although the results are not all consistent, it seems that the carboxyhaemoglobin in red cells does not correlate with changes in filterability. Therefore if there is a decreased filterability with cigarette smoking it is perhaps not due to carboxyhaemoglobin.

P.G. Professor Forconi will give the next presentation on myocardial and leg ischaemia.

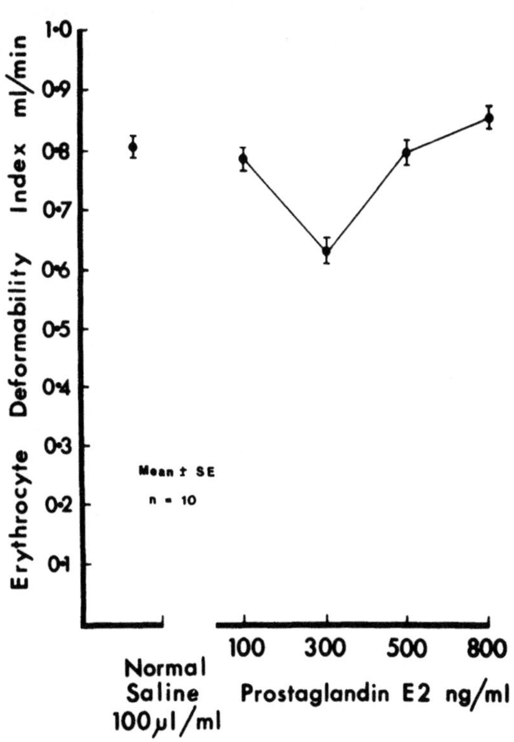

Fig. 7.16

S.F. The interrelationship between red cell deformability and peripheral ischaemia has interested us for several years. In these studies we evaluated red cell deformability using the whole blood filtration technique since we believe that the deformability of the red cell is the most important determinant of the filterability index. You must forgive me if most of you have already seen these slides on other occasions. In my first slide (Fig. 7.17) you can see the changes in red cell filterability in different groups of patients with circulatory disease. By comparison to controls patients with diabetes, peripheral obliterative arterial disease, atherosclerosis in the chronic stage and arterial hypertension all show a significant impairment of red cell filterability. The red cell filterability is correlated to the other rheological parameters such as blood, plasma and serum viscosity, haematocrit and fibrinogen concentration that in current rheological studies must be always investigated along with filterability.

The impression that filterability of red cells can change acutely and rapidly was enforced by our study of myocardial infarction. The lowest values for red cell filterability as well as the highest whole blood viscosity were recorded eight hours after the onset of symptoms. The close connection between red cell filterability and ischaemia is also well illustrated in this favourite slide of ours (Fig. 7.18). It shows the very rapid changes in red cell filterability with each attack of pain in one of our first patients with Prinzmetal angina. The red cell filterability can rapidly change even in a very few minutes during myocardial ischaemia.

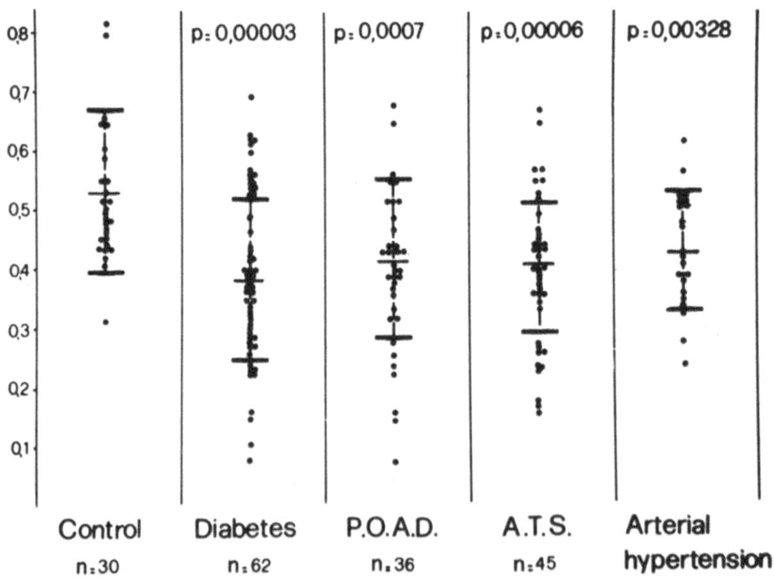

Fig. 7.17

Similarly with ischaemia provoking diagnostic procedures such as Master's test. Again there is no change in the red cell filterability of the controls but a significant decrease during pain brought on by ischaemic exercise. We also sampled blood directly from the coronary sinus during diagnostic atrial pacing. Again there was a significant decrease in red cell filterability before pacing and after pacing only in patients who developed pain. The general pattern is similar in peripheral ischaemic disease. Red cell filterability is already impaired under basal conditions and decreases further during pain induced by claudication. This slide (Fig. 7.20) summarises the percentage change with exercise in controls, coronary patients and peripheral arterial patients. In this study of a group of patients with severe peripheral obliterative arterial disease (Fig. 7.21) we showed that the femoral arterio-venous difference in red cell filterability was much greater in patients than in controls. These kinds of results led us to believe that red cell filterability is an important accompaniment of ischaemia and is both a diagnostic and a prognostic indicator. More importantly it is also a risk factor for the progression of vascular disease.

In a group of 80 patients with peripheral obliterative arterial disease we looked at the incidence of a number of haematological, biochemical and clinical parameters which are considered as risk factors (Fig. 7.22). Impaired red cell filterability was present in 92% of cases and was the commonest abnormality. When we analysed this data in terms of the severity of the peripheral ischaemia we again

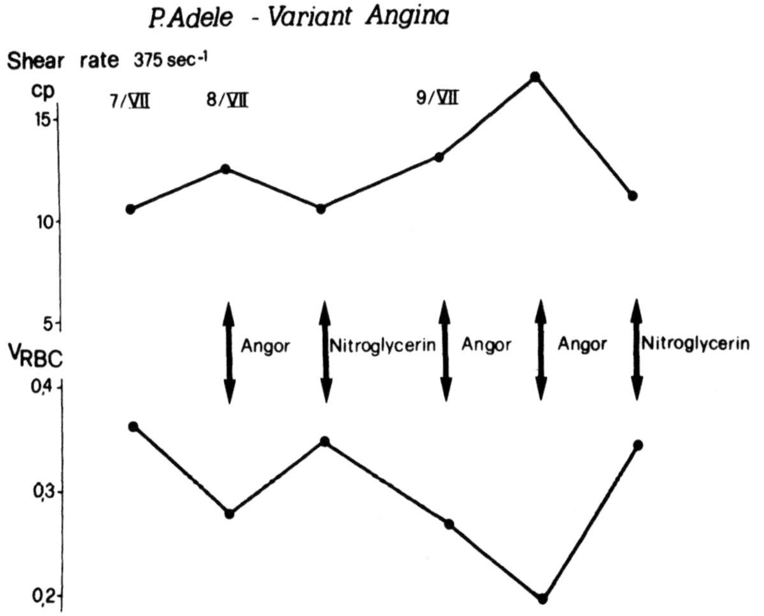

Fig. 7.18

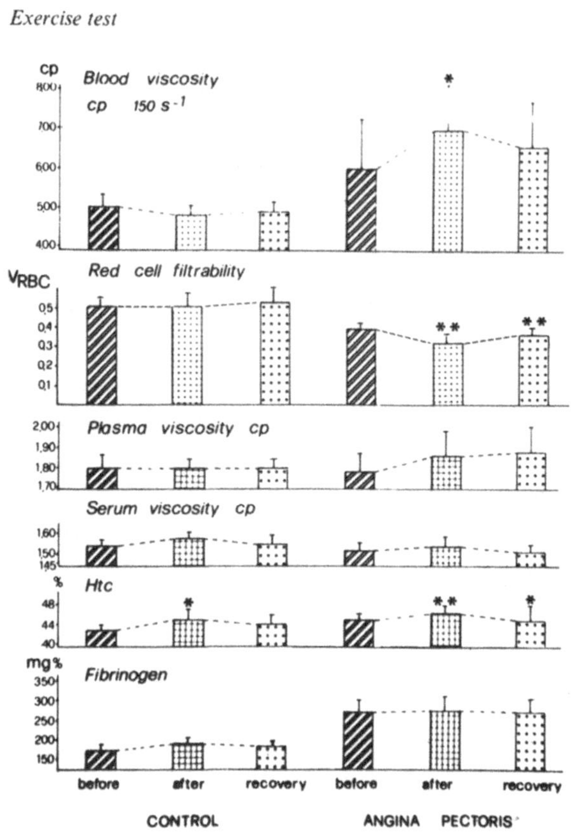

Fig. 7.19

found that the best correlation was obtained with red cell filterability.

These concepts lead us to consider the opportunity of treating ischaemic disease with substances capable of improving red cell deformability. Here some drugs are listed with their own rheological peculiarities according to our experience (Fig. 7.23). The differences in administration, activity and ability to improve the rheological parameters (blood flow in the legs included) are also shown.

In this slide (Fig. 7.24), we consider the effect of normovolemic haemodilution, an up-to-date procedure suggested by many authors for the treatment of ischaemic patients. As you can see, with a daily haemodilution (300 ml the first day, 150 ml from the second to the seventh day, using dextran 40 immediately infused after the blood withdrawal) we could observe a reduction of blood viscosity and of the haematocrit; but on the other hand, there was a significant

Exercise test (% changes)

	Control	Coronary artery disease	Peripheral artery disease
Whole blood viscosity (shear rate 150 sec^{-1})	−3,4	+16	+23
Plasma viscosity (shear rate 375 sec^{-1})	—	+4,5	+7,5
Serum viscosity (shear rate 375 sec^{-1})	+2,5	+3,3	+1,8
Htc	+4,6	+4	+4,4
V_{RBC}	+0,4	−19	−36
Plasma fibrinogen	+7,7	+3,3	+2,8
Plasma osmolality	+0,7	+1	+1

Fig. 7.20

Femoral A.V. differences (% changes)

	Control	Peripheral artery disease
Whole blood viscosity (shear rate 150 sec^{-1})	+1,9	+19,5
Plasma viscosity (shear rate 375 sec^{-1})	+3,5	+3
Serum viscosity (shear rate 375 sec^{-1})	+3,2	+2,5
Htc	+2	+4
Plasma fibrinogen	+1	+1
V_{RBC}	−3,4	−15,7

Fig. 7.21

Parameters studied with relative incidence %

	P	BL		P	BL
Red cell filtrability	92		Triglycerides	31	18
Blood viscosity	68.5	6.2	Uric acid	28	22
Tot. chol./Hdl chol. ratio	68.5	1.8	Total cholesterol	18	25
Smoking	68	12	Systolic blood pressure	16	14
Plasma viscosity	60	23.7	Diastolic blood pressure	15	10
Serum viscosity	52.5	23.7	Total lipemia	13.9	23.8
Hdl Cholesterol	39.8	9.2	Haematocrit	12.5	15
Diabetes	36		Fibrinogen	6.2	21.2

Fig. 7.22

Differences in rheological activity of some drugs

Drug	Isox-suprine	Cinnari-zine	Flunari-zine	Pentoxi-filline	Nicer-goline	Buflomedil
Administration						
Parenteral	Yes	No	No	Yes	Yes	Yes
Per os	Yes	Yes	Yes	Yes	Yes	Yes
Activity						
In vitro	Yes	?	?	Yes	?	No
In vivo	Yes	Yes	Yes	Yes	Yes	Yes
Improves						
Blood viscosity	Yes	Yes	Yes	Yes	Yes	No
Plasma viscosity	Yes	No	No	No	No	No
Serum viscosity	Yes	No	No	No	No	No
Haematocrit	Yes	No	No	No	Yes	No
Fibrinogen	Yes	No	Si	No	No	No
Red cell deformability	No	Yes	Yes	Yes	Yes	Yes*
Blood flow	Yes	Yes	Yes	Yes	No	No
Platelet aggregability	Yes	No	No	Yes	Yes	Yes

* Protective activity against the exercise-induced reduction of red cell deformability of vascular patients

Fig. 7.23

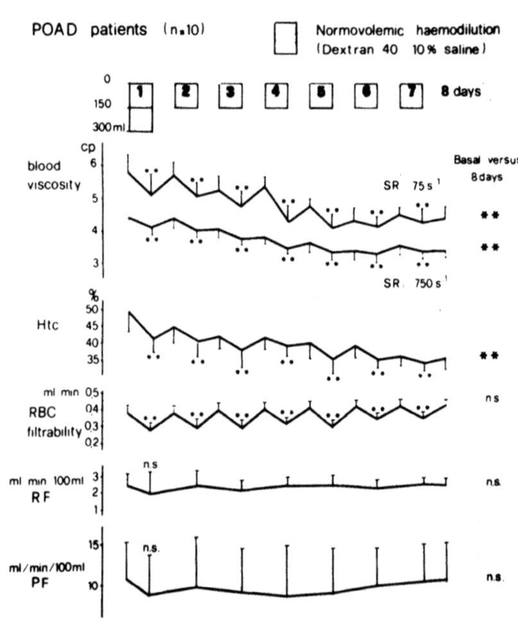

Fig. 7.24

decrease of red cell filterability and there was no effect on the blood flow of the legs, whether at rest (RF) or during reactive hyperemia (PF). Consequently we are doubtful about the effectiveness of this therapeutic procedure.

P.G. And now we will hear John Dormandy on the same topic.

J.D. I want to rapidly present some data on peripheral vascular disease and myocardial infarction which illustrates the kind of longitudinal study where patients are followed clinically after the haemorheological measurements have been made. As far as ischaemia in the leg is concerned, our latest and most long-term data are shown in the first two slides (Figs. 7.25 and 7.26). There is a significant difference in the red cell filtration of a group of claudicants compared to matched controls. Filtration, under gravity only, was carried out on red cells resuspended at a concentration of 5% in pre-filtered plasma after removing the buffy coat. We evaluated the progress of these patients for a minimum of a year after the measurements in terms of clinical course, whether they required vascular reconstruction or ultimately amputation. Within the claudicant group, smoking, age and diabetes could not be related to the reduction in red cell filtration. However, the ankle to arm pressure ratio, clinical deterioration, the

Statistical data of RCF

	Claudicants	Controls
n	88	66
$\bar{x}$	0.43	0.58
SD	0.10	0.09

$t = -8.82$; $p < 0.001$

Fig. 7.25

No significant reduction in RCF compared to matched patients

- Smoking
- Age
- Diabetes

Significant reduction in RCF compared to matched patients

	n	Change	p
– pressure indexes < 100 mm Hg	13	–23%	>0.001
– clinical deterioration	15	–13%	<0.05
– subsequent vascular surgery	12	–10%	<0.05
– subsequent amputation	8	–23%	<0.01

Fig. 7.26

need for subsequent vascular surgery and most importantly probably the need for amputation in the subsequent follow-up period were correlated with a decreased red cell filterability index in this prospective study. Our results in myocardial infarction have been published (Fig. 7.27). Like Forconi we found a very low red cell filterability within the first 12 hours after the onset of chest pain. There was a very good correlation between the initial red cell filterability and the subsequent development of pulmonary oedema and cardiogenic shock. When we looked at all the other data normally measured in patients with suspected myocardial infarction, such as enzyme changes, the earliest and the best predictor of subsequent development of complications was the red cell filterability.

Fig. 7.28 attempts to summarise some of the literature on red cell filtration in myocardial ischaemia and leg ischaemia. I quote the first author and the year the information became available, and the number of patients studied. The technique of filtration used is only an approximation. A is the original technique of whole blood filtration at approximately a constant pressure, B indicates the same except that the red cells are washed and resuspended in a buffer, C is any constant flow system usually in a buffer and D is the recent technique where we use a 5%

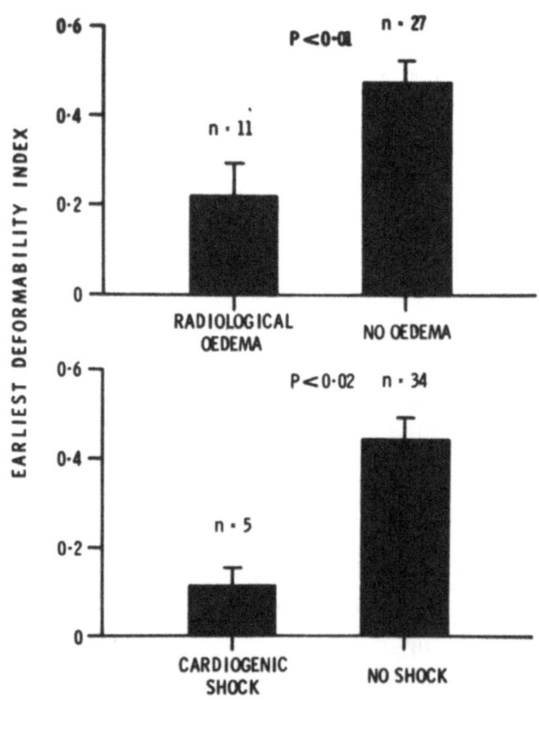

Fig. 7.27

n	RCF technique	Change cf. controls	Comments	Authors
Myocardial ischaemia				
26	—	– ?%	Acute – Prognostic	Volger *et al.*, 1979
15	A	– 14%	Acute	Drummond *et al.*, 1980
51	D	– 30%	Acute – Prognostic	Dormandy 1980 & 1981
12	A	– 25%	Chronic	Di Perri *et al.*, 1981
16	C	– 30%	Non-coronary angina	Johnson *et al.*, 1981
15		– ?%	Non-coronary angina	Cristal 1982
Leg ischaemia				
44	A	– 30%	Prognostic	Reid *et al.*, 1976
15	A	– 15%		Drummond *et al.*, 1980
25	A	– 35%		Angelkort et al., 1979
88	DD	– 35%	Prognostic	Ernst *et al.*, 1981
80	A	– 30%	Prognostic	Di Perri *et al.*, 1981
45	A	– 20%		Perego *et al.*, 1981
68	A	– 30%	Abolished by WBC corr	Alderman *et al.*, 1981
43	B, D	– 10%	Due to plasma	Winkenwerder *et al.*, 1982
11	A, D	– 15%		Juhan *et al.*, 1982
10	A, D	– 50%		Delauney *et al.*, 1982
—	C	N.S.		Stuart *et al.*, 1982

Fig. 7.28

suspension of red cells in pre-filtered plasma with the buffy coat removed. There seem to have been two studies in which there was a clear link between red cell filterability and subsequent clinical progress of a patient after myocardial ischaemia. In terms of leg ischaemia there were two prognostic studies plus what we have just heard from Professor Forconi. What is interesting, and you will also find this later on looking at other groups of patients, is that the mean change compared to the controls, which I have tried to estimate, is remarkably similar in all these different studies, about 20 to 30%. The other two studies I would like to draw your attention to are those by Dr Johnsson, which we heard last year in London, and by Professor Cristal, which is about to be published. Both studied subjects with so-called non-coronary angina, where the patients have all the symptoms and signs of myocardial infarction including abnormal ECG changes but in whom the coronary angiograms are normal. So these patients appear to have ischaemia without any arterial disease and in studies a considerable decrease in red cell filterability was found. Thank you very much.

P.G. Questions? Comments?

J.S. Is the predictive value of the RCF any greater than that obtained by measuring plasma viscosity in the same patients?

J.D. Yes, it is better. I did not mention that in relation to the peripheral vascular patients, but our findings are the same as Professor Forconi's; in terms of prediction of progress there is no other laboratory measurement that is equally reliable.

G.L. A comment about a recent study of many thousands of patients who have had a myocardial infarction and were followed up for several years to look for risk factors published recently in *Circulation*. Almost everything that can be measured was, apart from red cell filterability which was not invented when this project started, when they then performed a multivariate analysis of all the laboratory and clinical data, the white cell count emerged as the highest ranking blood test for predicting prognosis. So perhaps it is the white cell effect certainly in the whole blood filtration tests, and possibly also more than we like to think in the other tests, which makes the results clinically significant.

J.S. Is it perhaps just a question of which is the most sensitive test to detect the acute phase or the chronic phase response in these patients? Is it more sensitive to count the white cells, or suspend red cells in plasma and place them in an ESR tube, or to take red cells and put them in their plasma and filter them, or measure plasma proteins, or collectively measure plasma proteins as the plasma viscosity? All we are doing is measuring the acute or chronic phase response by a variety of different techniques, and the question is which is the most sensitive for picking up protein changes and their interaction with red cells.

J.D. I would have thought that you would have to distinguish between acute and chronic reactions. In the acute situations the changes in red cell filterability are extraordinarily rapid as you saw in many of the previous presentations, they can occur within minutes. But the protein changes take days or at least hours to occur.

J.S. You can only say that if you know exactly when the acute phenomenon started.

J.D. Professor Forconi did, because he induced many of the acute events.

S.F. I want to ask an opinion from John Dormandy. What is your opinion about non-coronary angina? Is it possible to explain it only in terms of haemorheology?

J.D. I am no expert on cardiology, but it would seem perfectly conceivable that a haemorheological change plays a primary role.

P.G. Now Tony Marcel is due to give his presentation on the pharmacological aspects of red cell filtration.

G.A.M. The first thing the pharmacologist has to ask for is a pharmacological exploration of the phenomenon of red cell filtration, which is more or less the same as a physiological one. I will not go through the indirect methods of testing except to mention the importance of assessing osmotic fragility, changes in mean cell volume and inhibition of crenation induced by calcium and ionophores. Even though we are working on red cell filterability we have to check that we are not incidentally making the red cell dangerously fragile, too large or too small. Of course, tests of new pharmacological agents must be made *ex vivo* and *in vitro*, both in normals and in diseased people. *In vitro* there is a great need for sensitised test or stress tests as some people call them. The exercise stress test Professor Forconi has talked about is one of the most recent and most exciting tests in clinical pharmacology of haemorheology. The fact that certain patients with peripheral ischaemic disease will have decreased filterability only after a certain amount of exercise is very important and of course you can check influence of various drugs on this effect as Professor Forconi has. You must always check that the dose used in the test has some analogy with the recommended dose for patients or else you can find some very strange reports in certain papers. Similarly, not only must results be significant but they must be performed double blind and if the drug improves filterability for instance in peripheral arterial disease by 30% we must remember that regular exercise and walking will do exactly the same. As for conditions of testing are concerned, the duration of incubation *in vitro* of the drug and the red cells is particularly important; certain drugs need a two-hour incubation to have a clearcut effect, others will have an immediate effect. We know that if we want to get calcium into the cell we practically have to incubate it for more than two hours. I would like to detail two further considerations, the pore length and the calcium problem. It is interesting to note that pentoxyfiline is usually active at 10^{-4} M using the Reid-Dormandy method and 10^{-6} M in the single pore erythrocyte rigidometer. As Dr Teitel has pointed out to us, this can of course be related to the differences of shear stress. If the pore is ten times longer, then of course the shear stress will be ten times smaller, which may be the explanation of the difference in efficacy. It might be interesting when rating efficacy of a drug on red cells to state at what shear stress precisely this has been measured. Another problem is the calcium problem. We all know that the intracellular erythrocyte concentration of calcium is about 100 times smaller than in plasma and that in certain cases plasma calcium has a nasty tendency to go inside the red cells. We compared red cells incubated in various concentrations of calcium either with saline or with pentoxyfiline (Fig. 7.29) and it is interesting to see that whether you use a medium with 4 mmol calcium, 2.5 mmol calcium or no calcium at all, the action is the same. So you can say that here the action is not calcium dependent and I think that is interesting because we might be coming to one of the first classifications of drugs acting on microfiltration: drugs without calcium antagonistic effect like pentoxyfiline and drugs with calcium antagonistic actions. All this leads me to this sort of table I try using when evaluating a drug (Fig. 7.30).

Red cells can be sensitised by storage for varying times at various temperatures, pH or osmolality. They can be heat treated or glutaraldehyde treated. Then you have got to see what the filtration test does either at constant pressure using the Reid-Dormandy derived tests, the haemorheometer or Hanss' apparatus, the filtrometer and the single pore erythrocyte rigidometer. Alternatively you can choose one of the constant flow tests, either measuring total

Efficacy of Pentoxifylline (7.10^{-4} M) in reducing the Hanss Time Filtration Index (TFI) or a constant flow Pressure Filtration Index (PFI), whatever the calcium concentration.

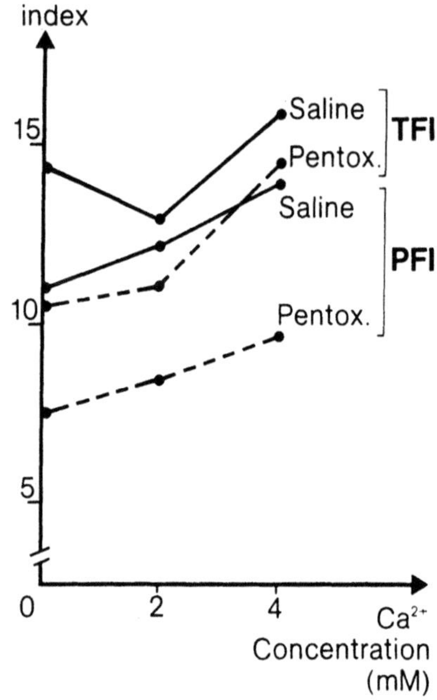

Fig. 7.29

change or just the very fast initial variation in pressure as has been suggested by Chien and Skalak. It is important also to have some data on viscometry, at high and low shear rates so as not to miss some new phenomena. I do not know how important it is to check for an effect on thixotropy and viscoelasticity. I have not read any clearcut and very exciting results obtained by ektacytometry as compared to results obtained by other simpler methods.

A table reviewing the effects of drugs on haemorheology is reproduced here. I think it is interesting to note that many great anti-aggregant agents do not act on red cell filterability. There is here in this room a great concentration of people concerned with these findings: I think that about 70% of what is known about the pharmacology of red cell deformability has been described by participants of this group. All I would like to add is that we have a great responsibility in our hands and must be very careful about what we write. It is easy to put in a paper that a drug increases red cell filterability, we all know that that is quite different from 'has an action on filterability', and I think especially now we know that this is different it must be put very clearly in the various papers.

One last word, it is getting more and more impossible to work in this field without being confronted by sickle cell disease. Amongst the drugs possibly acting on sickle cell disease, I think we can distinguish four families. The inhibitors of gelation, the drugs which lower the quantity of sickling haemoglobin,

	Red cells: (in-vitro or ex-vivo)							
		Sensitised cells						
	Normal cells	Disease	Conservation	Decreased pH	Osmolality	Increased heat	Glutaraldehyde	Diamide
FILTRATION TESTS								
Constant pressure								
Reid et Dormandy								
• whole blood								
• cells suspended in plasma								
• cells suspended in buffer								
Haemorheometer (Hanss)								
Filtrometer (Teitel)								
Single erythrocyte rigidometer								
Constant flow								
VISCOMETRY								
Stationary								
Blood a) high shear rate								
b) low shear rate								
Plasma								
Non stationary								
Influence on thixotropy								
Viscoelasticity								
Ektacytometry								
OTHER METHODS								
Centrifugation (Sirs)								
Osmotic resistance								
M.C.V.								
Crenation induced by Calcium								

Fig. 7.30

the drugs which act directly on the red cell membrane and the drugs which could inhibit adhesion of sickle cells to endothelial cells without doing anything else. A first point concerns pharmacological tests of gelation inhibitors. Some drugs show an increase of the delay time before the beginning of gelation which is important, but do not show a modification of the saturating concentration. Now, it is important to have both results and both should be assessed. There are quite a few drugs which seem to have a certain amount of clinical efficacy in sickle cell disease. I would just like to quote Briehl because he certainly knows

Haemorheological effects of some pharmacological agents

	Aspirin	Bencyclane	Buflomedil	Cinnarizine	Dipyridamole	Flunarizine	Isoxsuprine	Naftidrofuryl	Pentoxifylline	Suloctidil	Ticlopidine
FILTERABILITY DEFORMABILITY *Constant pressure* Reid et Dormandy									■●◆ 23, 24, 30, 31, 35, 36, 37, 38, 39, 40, 44		
• whole blood	○ 11	● 16	● 47		○ 22					○ 14	○ 10
• resuspended in plasma			● 17			● 3			■ 29		
• resuspended in buffer (also haemorheometer or filtrometer techniques)									■ 27, 33, 34		
Constant flow (including single erythrocyte rigidometer)									■● 25, 28, 32, 41, 46		
WHOLE BLOOD VISCOSITY Shear rate above 10 sec^{-1}			● 47	● 5			● 8	● 19	■○ 29, 47, 49, 50	● 14	
Shear rate below 10 sec^{-1}	● 12	● 48		● 5			● 8	● 19	● 47	● 14	

Significant results: ■ in vitro; ● in vivo; ◆ double blind; ○ no change.

Note: the numbers refer to the numbered special referencelist, at the end of this chapter, p. 214.

Fig. 7.31

this better than I do: 'A 1% change in Csat, which might not be easily picked up, will induce an increase in delay time of over 50%'.

Another important point concerns the lowering of deoxyhaemoglobin concentration and the 2-3DPG problem. We know that the SS red cells will sickle normally at 40 mm of mercury and AS would sickle at 15. If you increase 2-3DPG the curve will go towards the right, and that means that your SS haemoglobin will sickle at 45 mm of mercury instead of 40. So one might say let us decrease 2-3DPG but Murayama and colleagues have pointed out that if you decrease 2-3DPG too much you may not sickle any more but you will not deliver any oxygen. On the other hand, it is important to know from the pharmacological point of view that practically every vasodilator increases 2-3DPG, therefore they can have a two-sided effect, advantage and inconvenience. Thank you.

P.L. I want to just say a word about 2-3DPG and point out that these sickler patients being all anaemic probably already have a right shift to their curve so that it would not be much of a problem in terms of oxygen delivery to think of moving the curve back to the left, contrary to what you said.

P.G. Thank you. I think it is now John's task to say a few concluding words.

J.D. I want to deal with this in two ways. First of all going through the various groups of diseases as we did just now and then briefly looking at them in relation to the five criteria which I suggested in my introduction. I have already shown some of the published evidence as far as myocardial and leg ischaemia is concerned. We have heard from Professor Stuart that red cell filterability certainly does have clinical relevance in sickle cell disease and particularly interesting are the two patients whose blood happen to have been measured before their crises. In addition we have heard from Paul Teitel that there was a decreased red cell filterability in many classical haematological states and this of course is of obvious clinical relevance.

Fig. 7.32 summarises the data in relation to diabetes, and there seems to be a

Diabetes n	RCF technique	Change cf. controls	Comments	Authors
—	A	– ?%	Millipore filters	Ditzel *et al.*, 1970
77	B	–20%	Related to control	Schmid-Schönbein *et al.*, 1976
64	A	–20%	Related to retinopathy	Barnes *et al.*, 1977
—	A	– ?%		Ehrly *et al.*, 1977
12%	A, B	–25%	Related to insulin	Juhan *et al.*, 1981
62	A	–25%		Di Perri *et al.*, 1981
157	A	–30%	Related to control	Volger *et al.*, 1981
37	A	–40%	Related to complications	Pozza *et al.*, 1981
50	B	–30%	Related to complications	Delobel *et al.*, 1981
69	A	–30%	Related to complications	Diamantopoulos *et al.*, 1981
57		– ?%	Related to retinopathy	Palareti *et al.*, 1981
42	B	N.S.		Rand *et al.*, 1981
331	A	– ?%	Trial not completed	Hanss *et al.*, 1982
	A	–15%	PROGNOSTIC	Le Devehat *et al.*, 1982
22	C	– ?%	Related to control	Lowe *et al.*, 1982

Fig. 7.32

little doubt that red cell filterability measured by any method is related to diabetic control and most people seem to feel that it is related to the development of complications. We have not heard unfortunately the very interesting data which we have read through, from Dr Juhan, about the effect of red cell filterability on platelet aggregation which is obviously of considerable clinical relevance but was not dealt with during this session.

Now if we go on to the next slide (Fig. 7.33). These are the various trials in relation to cardiovascular risk factors, smoking and hypertension. Another area we did not really talk about is summarised in the next slide (Fig. 7.34).

Amongst the studies on cerebrovascular circulation we now have two studies where red cell filterability was found to have prognostic significance. And the last slide in this group (Fig. 7.35) are miscellaneous conditions including neonatal jaundice, where the evidence is almost the best in terms of clinical significance.

Altogether I find there are approximately 50 reports showing a clinical correlation between red cell filterability and various circulatory diseases. It is interesting that the kind of mean differences people describe between the patients and control seem to fall within the 20 to 40% bracket. Professor Chien's comment may be relevant that if the change in red cell filterability is very great then one might possibly loose that effect with some techniques of measurement where it would be interpreted as a white cell.

If we now consider the five criteria of clinical relevance that I mentioned at the beginning, as far as the first one is concerned, we have the two patients with sickle cell crisis, we have two studies where there was a correlation between red cell filterability and myocardial ischaemia in the absence of any coronary disease.

n	RCF technique	Change cf. controls	Comments	Authors
Cardiovascular risk factors				
72	A	−25%		Lagrue *et al.*, 1979
80	A	−30%		Lorient *et al.*, 1979
—	—			Stoltz 1981
Smoking				
11	A	−11%	Only in acute smoking	Drummond *et al.*, 1979
65	A	−12%	Acute and chronic	Lagrue *et al.*, 1979
10	B	−15%	Chronic	Rand *et al.*, 1981
9	B	−20%	Chronic	Norton *et al.*, 1981
60	—	N.S.		Landgraf *et al.*, 1981
Hypertension				
21	A	−25%		Di Perri *et al.*, 1981
28	A	− ?%	Essential hypertension	Palareti *et al.*, 1981

Fig. 7.33

Cerebrovascular disease

n	RCF technique	Change cf. controls	Comments	Authors
—	—	− ?%		Yoritsune 1978
—	—	− ?%		Takahashi 1978
49	A	−100%	Recent CVA	Martin *et al.*, 1979
80	A	− 60%	Recent CVA	Lorient *et al.*, 1979
—	—	− ?%	Old CVA	Yamamoto *et al.*, 1981
102	A	− ?%	Old CVA	Coccheri *et al.*, 1981
55	A	− ?%	CVA	Ott *et al.*, 1981
			CVA – Prognostic	Boisseau *et al.*, 1981
10	A	− ?%	Recent CVA	Guerrini *et al.*, 1981
26	A, B	N.S.		Pollack *et al.*, 1981
	A	− ?%	CVA – Prognostic	Deshayes *et al.*, 1982

Fig. 7.34

The study by Palaretti showing decreased red cell filterability in essential hypertension could well be related to aetiology of that disease. And today we just heard about oxcytocin and neonatal jaundice which would also come under that first heading. Going on to the second criterion, a possible role in the pathophysiological process characteristic of the disease, the majority of the clinical studies I listed fall into this group, particularly in relation to diabetic microangiopathy, Raynaud's and cerebral ischaemia. The results shown by Sandro Forconi, that the changes in filterability of the red cells associated with a physiological stress like exercise is different in patients who suffer from ischaemic disease than in normals, is extremely interesting and well worth pursuing. The third criterion was an indication of the incidence of severity of complications. Again there is a considerable body of evidence in relation to diabetes, ischaemia of the legs and myocardial ischaemia. In some of these it is compared to other prognostic factors and red cell filterability has been found to be a better prognostic indicator than anything else. With regard to prognosis we have two studies on myocardial ischaemia, two on intermittent claudication, two on cerebrovascular disease and possibly you could consider the papers relating to cardiovascular risk factors. All these six or seven studies seem to show that changes in red cell filterability, whatever they measure, can be related to prognosis and in some cases it is the best or earliest prognostic indicator. And finally, most importantly from the clinical point of view, is the possibility that these studies help in the development of new forms of treatment and that of course was summarised in the last presentation by Dr Marcel.

P.G. Thank you, John. We now move on to the last session and Professor Chien is going to give a summary of specific recommendations for filtration tests.

n	RCF technique	Change cf. controls	Comments	Authors
Stored blood				
6	B	– ?%		Haradin *et al.*, 1969
14	B	– ?%	RCF diminished after 3 litres	Scholtz *et al.*, 1975
16	D	– ?%	RCF diminished after 3 litres	Dodds *et al.*, 1980
	A	– ?%		Quemada *et al.*, 1982
Deep venous thrombosis				
63	A	N.S.	No predictive value	Lowe *et al.*, 1982
Oral contraceptives				
34	B	–50%		Oski *et al.*, 1972
38	C	–20%		Buchan *et al.*, 1980
9	A	–20%	Only severe pre-eclampsia	Thorburn *et al.*, 1982
Pre-eclampsia				
120	C	– ?%		Buchan *et al.*, 1981
Chronic renal failure				
21	B	–90%	Only if splenectomised (n = 7)	Forman *et al.*, 1973
23	—	– ?%		Rosemund *et al.*, 1975
—	B	– ?%	Improved by dialysis	Droulle 1982
Alcoholic liver failure				
120	—	– ?%		Gueguen *et al.*, 1981
Raynaud's phenomenon				
8	D	–50%	Improved by plasma-pheresis	Dodds *et al.*, 1979
—	A	–50%		Dowd *et al.*, 1981
Burns				
—	A	– ?%	Related to area of burn at one to two months	Guimbretiere *et al.*, 1980

Fig. 7.35

References to Fig. 7.31

1. F. De Clerck, et al. Arch. int. Pharmacodyn., 1977, *230*: 321–323.
2. F. De Clerck, et al. In Hemorheology and diseases; Stoltz J.F., Drouin P. Eds: 669–676; Doin Editeurs, 1980.
3. J. De Cree, et al. Angiology, 1979, *30*: 505–515.
4. C. K. Scott, et al. Angiology, 1980, *31*: 320–330.
5. T. Di Perri, et al. Proc. Roy. Soc. Med., 1978, *70* (Suppl. 8): 25–28.
6. M. Guerrini, et al. 2nd European Conference on Clinical Haemorheology, 30 Sept. – 2 Oct., London 1981, abstract n° 226.

7. A.M. Ehrly, et al. 2nd European Conference on Clinical Haemorheology, 30 Sept. – 2 Oct., London 1981, abstract n° 185.
8. T. Di Perri, et al. Br. J. Clin. Pharmac., 1978, *5*: 255–260.
9. T. Di Perri, et al. Angiology, 1981, *32*: 257–265.
10. S. Ono, et al. Thromb. Haemost., 1981, *46*, abstract n° 0544.
11. M. Stäubli, et al. Atherosclerosis, 1982, *41*: 167–170.
12. R. Bonniot, et al. Archives Médicales de l'Ouest, 1980, *12*: 577–594.
13. M. Gueguen, et al. Le Praticien, 1981, *376*: 57–64.
14. R. Roncucci, et al. Arzneim. Forsch./Drug Res., 1979, *29* (I), Nr. 4.
15. P. Chatelain, et al. Biochemical Pharmacology, *30*: 313–317.
16. C. Le Devehat, et al. Angéiologie XXXII, 1980, *4*: 177–181.
17. J.A. Dormandy, et al. Angiology, 1981, *32*: 714–716.
18. M. Materazzi, et al. 2nd European Conference on Clinical Haemorheology, 30 Sept. – 2 Oct., London 1981, Abstract n° 230.
19. L. Savi, et al. La Vie Médicale, 1979, *60*: 285–287.
20. J. Hudomel, et al. Ophtal. Res., 1977, *9*: 25–30.
21. R.L. Henry, et al. Diabetes, 1981, *30* (Suppl. 1), 83 A, abstract n° 330.
22. M. Harrison, et al. 2nd European Conference on Clinical Haemorheology, 30 Sept. – 2 Oct., London 1981, abstract n° 167.
23. A.M. Ehrly. IRCS Medical Science, 1975, *3*: 465.
24. U. Werner. Med. Welt., 1975, *26*: 2098–2099.
25. C. Vigneron, et al. Médecine Actuelle, 1977, *4*: 200–204.
26. M. Guillot, et al. Third Int. Congress of Biorheology, La Jolla, 28 Aug. – 1 Sept. 1978, abstract p. 150.
27. J.A. Dormandy, et al. Current Medical Research and Opinion, 1981, *7*: 520–522.
28. Y. Isogai, et al. Current Medical Research and Opinion, 1981, *7*: 352–358.
29. H. Leonhardt, et al. Naunyn-Schmiedeberg's Arch. Pharmacol, 1977, *299*: 197–200.
30. H. Leonhardt, et al. La Ricerca Clin. Lab., 1978, *8*: 65–71.
31. H.G. Grigoleit, et al. VASA, 1977, *6*: 274–278.
32. D. Seiffge, et al. Klin. Wochenschr., 1981, *59*: 1271–1272.
33. D. Seiffge. Scand. J. Clin. Lab. Invest., 1981, *41* (Suppl. 156): 251–253.
34. D. Seiffge, et al. La Ricerca Clin. Lab., 1981, *11* (Suppl. 1): 117–123.
35. J.A. Sirs, et al. Biorheology, 1978, *15*: 53–54.
36. P. Martin, et al. Current Medical Research and Opinion, 1980, *6*: 512–522.
37. C. Le Devehat, et al. Scand. J. Clin. Lab. Invest., 1981, *41* (Suppl. 156): 301–303.
38. S. Gaillard, et al. Annales Médicales de Nancy et de l'Est. 1979; *XVIII*: 1099–1102.
39. R. Schubotz, et al. Curr. Med. Res. Opin., 1977, *4*: 609–617.
40. B. Angelkort, et al. Curr. Med. Res. Opin., 1979, *6*: 255–258.
41. R. Johnsson, et al. Scand. J. Clin. Lab. Invest., 1981, *41* (Suppl. 156): 297–300.
42. H. Nagata, et al. 10th Europ. Conf. Microcirculation. Biblthca anat., N° 18, pp. 125–128 (Karger, Basel 1979).
43. K.I. Zinzadse, et al. Pharmatherapeutica, 1978, *2* (Suppl. 1): 118–122.
44. H.G. Grigoleit, et al. Pharmatherapeutica, 1976, *1*: 241–247.
45. D. Harwart. Current Medical Research and Opinion, 1979, *6*: 73–84.
46. D. Seiffge. In '7ème Réunion du Groupe Français de Filtration Erythrocytaire, !982, p. 21.
47. M.A. Perego, et al. Angéiologie *XXXIV*, 1982: 33–41.
48. B. Störmer, et al. Current Medical Research and Opinion, 1977, *4*: 588–595.
49. H. Heidrich, et al. IRCS Medical Science, 1976, *4*: 368.
50. H. Hess, et al. Fortschr. Med., 1973, *91*: 743–748.

SESSION 8

Specific recommendations for filtration tests

P.G. It was Professor Chien's task to present a summary on the assessment of the various recommendations for filtration tests.

S.C. We have had a very fruitful work group meeting on filtration. Many valuable recommendations have been made by the participants, and I will try to summarise them. On some of the points discussed we do not have unanimity in opinion. I am not sure that we should always have uniformity in the filtration procedure. On the one hand, for clinical tests it would be nice to have the same procedure so that we can compare the results from different groups; but on the other hand, in order to develop new approaches we must try different methods. It has also been mentioned that we should try various ways to sensitise or stress the cells, i.e. we should sometimes depart from a standard protocol. Therefore, while we want to unify the approaches in various laboratories, we should also allow for differences. I would divide my talk into four parts.

I. *The sampling procedure and sample preparation*

(a) Drawing of the sample: Professor Stuart talked in detail about the conditions of sampling, including patient preparation, time of the day, relation to meal and the drawing of the sample without a tourniquet. One point I would like to bring up again is the drawing of blood samples with a syringe versus the vacutainer. This needs to be tested with more definitive experiments so that we know whether we can use the vacutainer or not.

(b) Anticoagulants: There are suggestions of using large volume dilution so that we do not have to use anticoagulants, but this is not always possible because samples are usually taken in the wards into tubes containing anticoagulant. In terms of the relative merits of EDTA and heparin, we do not have a final conclusion, but probably for the time being it is better to use EDTA.

(c) White cells and platelets: We all agree that in order to derive red cell deformability from a filtration test we must try to remove the white cells as much as possible. The role of platelets is probably important,but they will be removed at the same time anyway by washing or prefiltration. Even after these procedures, it is advisable to measure the white cell concentration in the suspension to be filtered.

(d) The suspending medium: Some people use plasma, while others use various kinds of buffer. We should probably do both, particularly for clinical tests, but we must keep in mind that filterability of red cells in plasma is affected by red cell aggregation. When we study suspensions of red cells in buffer, it is necessary to control the osmolality and pH as well as to add glucose. Albumin ($\simeq 0.5\%$) is needed to maintain the normal cell shape; whether it is needed in filtration tests should be assessed critically. For cell suspension in plasma, if CO_2 is allowed to escape the pH would become more alkaline. We don't know whether this would affect the filterability test. Whatever buffer medium we use, we should pre-filter the medium. The pre-filtered buffer should be passed through the test filter in order to calculate the cell filterability and also to characterise the filter.

(e) Time delay: The time required for preparation and the delay between the preparation and measurement should be kept to a minimum. If we must store the sample, the whole blood should be stored at room temperature, not at 4° C; once the sample is diluted it should be measured as soon as possible. Of course, if we want to stress the sample we may purposely increase the delay time.

II. *The filter*

(a) The type of filter: Most investigators now use the Nuclepore polycarbonate filter, but we should also explore the possibility that other kinds of filters might yield additional information. For the time being, for standardisation it seems that the filter of choice is the Nuclepore filter, but that should not prevent us from comparing it with other kinds.

(b) Pore size: For standardisation probably the 5 μ filter is the most commonly used one, but we should not abandon the 3 μ because it may give information different from the 5 μ. We still do not have enough data to critically relate the two. The advantages of using the 5 μ over the 3 μ are a better reproducibility and a lesser possibility of haemolysis. With the 5 μ filter, one does not need as high a pressure gradient to drive the cells through, so the shear stress is lower than with 3 μ filters.

(c) Pore length: The usual standard polycarbonate filter has a pore length of approximately 12 μ. If we increase the pore length we can get a better flow condition in the filter. However, the entrance effect may be the predominant factor in the filtration tests. Therefore, it may be better to keep the pore length short; because the longer the pore, more of the resistance is due to the straight filtration through the pore rather than at the entrance. Of course, we should explore the effect of the pore length, so that we can evaluate how much is the entrance effect and how much is the dissipation in the pore itself.

(d) Pore density: Filters with very high density should be avoided, because there may be fusion of adjacent pores. Dr Leblond mentioned that there may be a problem with pore density, even at low density. That problem should also be investigated. In general, a relatively standard pore density such as about 10^5 pores per cm^2 should be fine with a 5 μ filter. The key is the quality control. Every time we must examine the pore size, determine the pore size distribution, the number of doublets, etc. In the publication we should report not only the nominal pore size and the batch number but also the measured pore size, perferably with a standard deviation. The pore size can be measured either by scanning electron microscopy or even by light microscopy, when using the 5 μ filters. Finally, we should pass the buffer through the filter and report the pressure–flow relationship, together with the pore density and the effective area of the filter that is exposed to the filtration process. By using these parameters and the viscosity of the buffer the effective mean pore density can be calculated from the Poiseuille-Hagen law. The result should agree within $\pm 10\%$ of the measured mean pore diameter.

III. *The filtration process*

(a) The time dependent behaviour: We all agree that there is a time-dependent behaviour in blood cell filtration and that the later phase of either the pressure tracing (at constant flow) or the flow tracing (at constant pressure) is due to either cell plugging or some very slowly moving cells affecting the curve. Therefore, in order to derive red cell deformability at constant pressure, we should take the initial flow, like in Dr Hanss' machine, or extrapolate back to 0 time, as Dr Dormandy does. At constant flow we should determine the initial pressure as in our studies at Columbia. Both of these approaches allow us to assess the filtration behaviour of the majority of the cells in the sample which is usually the red cells. By doing so we are losing the minority of cells, which may be less deformable, such as the white cells. But if one is interested in a small population of red cells these are more rigid than the majority of the red cells, the initial reading will not reflect the behaviour of these rigid cells.

(b) Comparison of the constant pressure and the constant flow methods: For the initial reading it really should not matter, but the behaviour of the later phase would differ between these two methods. Under constant flow the pressure will rise. For parallel pores the critical hydrodynamic parameter is the pressure drop rather than the flow; therefore the hydrodynamic condition changes with time in constant flow, but not in the constant pressure technique. Hence the constant pressure method provides a more stable hydrodynamic condition throughout the test.

(c) The shear stress: Very high shear stresses should be avoided because it would not allow the detection of minor changes in deformability. Furthermore, high shear stresses might cause haemolysis, particularly in the smaller pores. Dr Meiselman, however, purposely used the high stress to study the haemolysis and derived some information about red cell membrane. Nevertheless, the standard test should be performed at relatively low stresses, which may be more sensitive in detecting minor abnormalities; with a sledgehammer you can deform everything.

(d) Temperature: Most investigators perform their filtration test at room temperature without temperature control. But Forconi showed that temperature may be important. If possible, we should control the temperature, e.g. at 37° C.

(e) Filtration of buffer: The filtration procedure must be applied to the buffer in order to check the filter and also to calculate the relative resistance of the suspension to the buffer medium.

IV. *Calculation and expression of the results* (Fig. 8.1)

(a) The relative resistance: The resistance is the pressure–flow ratio (P/Q). In order to determine red cell properties from filtration data, we calculate the initial value of the relative resistance (R_{ri}), which is equal to the ratio of initial resistance of the suspension (R_i) to the resistance of the buffer (R_o)

$$R_{ri} = \frac{R_i}{R_o} = \frac{P_i/Q_i}{P_o/Q_o} = \frac{P_i\,Q_o}{P_o\,Q_i}$$

In the constant flow method, if the suspension and the buffer are subject to the same flow rate Q_c, then $R_{ri} = (\frac{P_i}{P_o})_{Q_c}$. In the constant pressure method, if the suspension and the buffer are filtered at the same pressure P_c, then $R_{ri} = (\frac{Q_o}{Q_i})_{P_c}$. Flow rate is equal to volume divided by time ($Q = V/t$). Therefore if the volumes filtered at a given constant pressure P_c over a given time period t_c are determined for the suspension and the buffer, then $R_{ri} = (\frac{V_o}{V_i})_{P_c, t_c}$. If the time periods taken to filter a given constant volume V_c at a given constant pressure P_c are determined for the suspension and the buffer, then $R_{ri} = (\frac{t_i}{t_o})_{P_c, V_c}$. Since the pressure–flow relationship for the buffer should be linear, it is not really necessary to run the filtration test at the same constant pressure level or (or the same constant flow level) for the buffer and the suspension, as long as appropriate correction is made.

Expression of results of filtration studies (initial values)

Initial resistance of suspension: $$R_i = \frac{P_i}{Q_i}$$

Resistance of suspending medium: $$R_o = \frac{P_o}{Q_o}$$

Initial relative resistance: $$R_{ri} = \frac{P_i/Q_i}{P_o/Q_o}$$

$$R_{ri} = \left(\frac{P_i}{P_o}\right)_{\text{const Q}} = \left(\frac{Q_o}{Q_i}\right)_{\text{const P}} = \left(\frac{t_i}{t_o}\right)_{\substack{\text{const P}\\ \text{const V}}} = \left(\frac{V_o}{V_i}\right)_{\substack{\text{const P}\\ \text{const t}}}$$

Intrinsic material properties of erythrocytes derived from filtration test (for the particular filter and filtration condition)

Additional Rigidity (or Resistance) due to a Single RBC in a Single Pore:

$$R_{ac} = \frac{R_{ri} - 1}{N_p}$$

where $N_p = \dfrac{H}{V_c/V_p}$,

H: Hematocrit/100, V_c: Mean Red Cell Volume, and V_p: Mean Pore Volume

RBC Rigidity Index (or RBC Resistance Index):

$$\text{R.I.} = 1 + R_{ac} = \frac{R_{ri} - 1}{N_p} + 1$$

RBC Filterability Index (or RBC Fluidity Index):

$$\text{F.I.} = \frac{1}{\text{R.I.}} = \frac{N_p}{R_{ri} - 1 + N_p}$$

Fig. 8.1

(b) The derivation of an expression of the intrinsic material properties of the red cell: The ultimate purpose of performing the filtration test is to derive the intrinsic material properties of the cells. It is obvious that the result will still depend upon the conditions of the experiment, e.g. the filter pore size and the flow condition. Therefore, the result represents a manifestation of the intrinsic material properties of the red cell under these experimental conditions.

The material properties can be expressed in terms of an index of the resistance for a single cell in a single pore in addition to that of the buffer (R_{ac}). $R_{ac} = \dfrac{R_{ri} - 1}{N_p}$ where N_p is the average number of red cells per pore; as Dr Skalak pointed out $N_p = \dfrac{H}{V_c/V_p}$ where H is the haematocrit in the feed suspension, V_c is the volume of the cell and V_p is the volume of the pore. In our studies on constant flow filtration through 5 μm pores, the value of R_{ac} for normal human red cells is between 2 and 3. In Dr Hanss' constant pressure filtration through 5 μm pores, he calculates the value of I.F. of about 10; I.F. is $(R_{ri} - 1)/H$ and hence equals R_{ac} (V_p/V_c). Since the value of V_p/V_c for 5 μm filters is about 0.3, his results would give a R_{ac} value of about 3, which is in agreement with our results, despite the differences in methodology and population studied. Therefore, R_{ac} is a manifestation of the material properties of red cells for a particular filter size (5 μm in these studies). If the red cells behave as the buffer, $R_{ri} = 1$ and R_{ac} becomes 0. If the cell becomes more rigid and gives rise to higher resistance, the value of R_{ac} increases. As pointed out above, R_{ac} is the additional resistance contributed by a red cell in a pore. We can also define an index of red cell resistance or red cell rigidity (RI) as $1 + R_{ac}$, i.e. the total resistance of a single red cell in a single pore.

$$\mathrm{RI} = R_{ac} + 1 = \frac{R_{\gamma i} - 1}{N_p} + 1$$

We may also express the results in terms of an index of filterability or fluidity (FI), which is the reciprocal of the index of resistance or rigidity.

$$\mathrm{FI} = \frac{1}{\mathrm{RI}} = \frac{1}{\dfrac{R_{\gamma i} - 1}{N_p} + 1} = \frac{N_p}{R_{\gamma i} - 1 + N_p}.$$

Since R_{ri} is greater than 1, RI is greater than 1 and FI is less than 1. As R_{ri} approaches the lower limit of 1, RI decreases toward 1 and FI rises toward 1.

The above are my suggestions with respect to the expression of the results of filtration studies. Regardless of what terminology we use, it is the concepts behind this that are more important. I think the emergence of these concepts is one of the major conclusions of the meeting, i.e. we have some way of obtaining an assessment of the intrinsic properties of the cell as a whole. An important aspect is how to apply such concepts to the clinical situation. I am very impressed by the way the various clinical investigations are carried out, I think many of the recommendations mentioned here have already been in practice.

Overall conclusions

P.G. This meeting has once more demonstrated that the 'simple' test of red cell filtration is indeed anything but simple. Much of its complexity results from the following three problems:

- the difficulty of providing the appropriate hydrodynamic test conditions which, on one hand, must be chosen so as to provide a 'mechanical challenge' to the cell without inducing 'mechanical damage'.
- the difficulty of defining those cellular properties which are actually being detected by the test. The discussion at this meeting has shown increasing agreement that the 'ease of entrance' into the pore rather than the cell passage through it influences the measurement. This certainly includes several aspects of red cell rheology such as elastic and viscous membrane properties or the viscosity of the intracellular hemoglobin; but it also includes morphological features of the cell such as surface area, volume, and shape.
- the difficulty of selecting appropriate conditions of the chemical environment (pH, anticoagulant, etc). Here, one faces the dilemma that conditions must to some extent be standardized if cellular properties only are to be measured, but in a standardized chemical environment alterations of these properties due to factors in the patient's own plasma may be masked.

We have again seen that many problems of filtration remain unsolved while others have become clearer. To me one of the most important remaining questions is that of relevance: Where and when do those red cell properties which are detected by filtration play a role, and what is, in quantitative terms, the importance of this role in physiology and in clinical situations? This needs further exploration obviously because of the clinical interest in red cell rheology which requires evaluation of the diagnostic and predictive value of red cell filtration.

It is now my task to try an assessment of the meeting. There are various ways of doing this: you could say a meeting is a good meeting when speakers have stayed within the time allowed, but you can also say it is a good meeting if the speakers have exceeded the time allowed. I lean towards the last definition and in this sense I think this has been an excellent meeting. You can also assess the performance of the moderator: there you can say a meeting has been good, if the moderator did not have a chance to say anything. In that sense it also was a good meeting. There is a third way of assessing the success of a meeting and that is by asking participants to express their views on what should be done in the future. This has been done: A vast majority of the participants voted in favour of having another meeting in one year's time. And the same majority was in favour of having the next meeting in London as opposed to any other place. Furthermore, a majority has voted in favour of slightly expanding the scope of the meeting. This, I think, is a difficult problem particularly in view of the comment made by Adrian Barnes, that the original reason for calling together a Working Group was to think about designing a simple test that can actually be used under clinical circumstances. If now the group says we want to expand our topics, then this could be interpreted to mean that either the participants have given up designing a simple test or they feel that this has already been achieved. The general opinion seems to be that we should take up the discussion of other methods in addition to filtration to assess deformability of red cells. The major thrust should be directed towards those methods which could be considered practical, clinically also.

I do not think I should close this meeting without expressing our sincere thanks to those who have actually organised the meeting: John Dormandy, Tony Marcel and Gordon Lowe.

GPSR Compliance

The European Union's (EU) General Product Safety Regulation (GPSR) is a set of rules that requires consumer products to be safe and our obligations to ensure this.

If you have any concerns about our products, you can contact us on ProductSafety@springernature.com

In case Publisher is established outside the EU, the EU authorized representative is:

Springer Nature Customer Service Center GmbH
Europaplatz 3
69115 Heidelberg, Germany

Batch number: 10607222

Printed by Printforce, the Netherlands